MRCOG Part-2
Single Best Answer Questions

MRCOG Part-2
Single Best Answer Questions
Extensive Revision Source

Shailaja Rao Puppala
MBBS MS MRCOG
Registrar
University Hospital
Coventry and Warwickshire NHS Trust, UK

Sushama Gupta
MBBS DGO MRCOG
Senior Registrar
Birmingham Women's and
Children's NHS Foundation Trust
Birmingham, UK

Foreword
Ruchira Singh

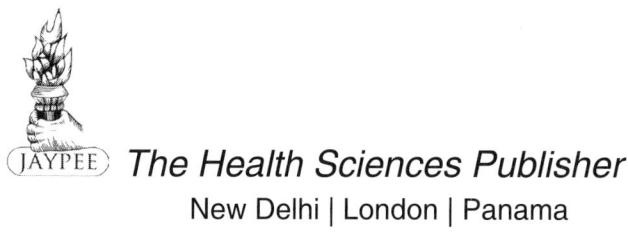

The Health Sciences Publisher
New Delhi | London | Panama

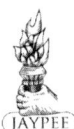
Jaypee Brothers Medical Publishers (P) Ltd

Headquarters
Jaypee Brothers Medical Publishers (P) Ltd
4838/24, Ansari Road, Daryaganj
New Delhi 110 002, India
Phone: +91-11-43574357
Fax: +91-11-43574314
Email: jaypee@jaypeebrothers.com

Overseas Offices

J.P. Medical Ltd
83 Victoria Street, London
SW1H 0HW (UK)
Phone: +44 20 3170 8910
Fax: +44 (0)20 3008 6180
Email: info@jpmedpub.com

Jaypee-Highlights Medical Publishers Inc
City of Knowledge, Bld. 235, 2nd Floor, Clayton
Panama City, Panama
Phone: +1 507-301-0496
Fax: +1 507-301-0499
Email: cservice@jphmedical.com

Jaypee Brothers Medical Publishers (P) Ltd
17/1-B Babar Road, Block-B, Shaymali
Mohammadpur, Dhaka-1207
Bangladesh
Mobile: +08801912003485
Email: jaypeedhaka@gmail.com

Jaypee Brothers Medical Publishers (P) Ltd
Bhotahity, Kathmandu
Nepal
Phone: +977-9741283608
Email: kathmandu@jaypeebrothers.com

Website: www.jaypeebrothers.com
Website: www.jaypeedigital.com

© 2018, Jaypee Brothers Medical Publishers

The views and opinions expressed in this book are solely those of the original contributor(s)/author(s) and do not necessarily represent those of editor(s) of the book.

All rights reserved. No part of this publication may be reproduced, stored or transmitted in any form or by any means, electronic, mechanical, photocopying, recording or otherwise, without the prior permission in writing of the publishers.

All brand names and product names used in this book are trade names, service marks, trademarks or registered trademarks of their respective owners. The publisher is not associated with any product or vendor mentioned in this book.

Medical knowledge and practice change constantly. This book is designed to provide accurate, authoritative information about the subject matter in question. However, readers are advised to check the most current information available on procedures included and check information from the manufacturer of each product to be administered, to verify the recommended dose, formula, method and duration of administration, adverse effects and contraindications. It is the responsibility of the practitioner to take all appropriate safety precautions. Neither the publisher nor the author(s)/editor(s) assume any liability for any injury and/or damage to persons or property arising from or related to use of material in this book.

This book is sold on the understanding that the publisher is not engaged in providing professional medical services. If such advice or services are required, the services of a competent medical professional should be sought.

Every effort has been made where necessary to contact holders of copyright to obtain permission to reproduce copyright material. If any have been inadvertently overlooked, the publisher will be pleased to make the necessary arrangements at the first opportunity. The **CD/DVD-ROM** (if any) provided in the sealed envelope with this book is complimentary and free of cost. **Not meant for sale.**

Inquiries for bulk sales may be solicited at: jaypee@jaypeebrothers.com

MRCOG Part-2 Single Best Answer Questions—Extensive Revision Source

First Edition: **2018**

ISBN: 978-93-5270-104-9

Printed at Sanat Printers

Foreword

This book is a valuable and comprehensive collection of *single best answer* (SBA) format for MRCOG part-2 examination. Preparing for the MRCOG exam is a difficult and daunting task for all the obstetricians and gynaecologists. The new format of the exam paper has been introduced in March 2015. There are two written papers in Part-2. Each paper consists of SBA questions worth 40% of the total mark and extended matching questions (EMQ) worth 60% of the total mark. Each paper consists of 50 SBAs and 50 EMQs to be completed in 180 minutes.

The MRCOG Part-2 examination is a clinical examination. From September, 2016, it consists of only written assessment and there is a separate Part-3 MRCOG for oral assessment. The candidates who are successful in MRCOG Part-2 must attempt the Part-3 MRCOG within 7 years. If they do not attempt the Part-3 MRCOG within this timeframe, they will be required to take up MRCOG Part-2 again.

The MRCOG Part-2 is blueprinted against a comprehensive syllabus which is available on the RCOG website. The MRCOG Part-2 examination incorporates what a standard ST5 level specialist registrar would be expected to do in managing patients in UK hospitals.

In preparation for MRCOG Part-2, the candidates should go through RCOG Green-top Guidelines, National Institute of Clinical Excellence (NICE) Guidelines, Good Practice Series and Scientific Papers from Royal College. With the introduction of SBAs, it is very important to broaden the knowledge by reading The Obstetrician and Gynaecologist (TOG) journals, Recent Advances in Obstetrics and Gynaecology by John Bonnar, all previous reports from MBRRACE-UK, Guidelines from Faculty of Sexual and Reproductive Healthcare (FSRH) and Scottish Intercollegiate Guidelines Network (SIGN).

This book attempts to cover the holistic nature of the exam, so that the candidates master the art of answering SBA questions.

Ruchira Singh
MD MRCOG
Consultant
Obstetrics and Gynaecology

Deputy Clinical Director
Birmingham Women's and Children's Hospital
Foundation Trust
UK

Preface

The *MRCOG Part-2* examination is mainly designed to test your application of clinical knowledge. Questions are presented as case scenarios that test your factual knowledge, understanding of latest clinical guidelines, research articles and systemic reviews.

This book is a great resource for single best answer (SBA) for candidates preparing to take up *MRCOG Part-2*. It has around 500 questions with explanation to answers and references along with further reading. In this book, we have tried to deal with SBA which has replaced multiple choice question (MCQ). A single best answer question typically has a stem describing the scenario with five plausible options, but clearly, there will be one correct answer. There has not been enough resources available to practice these questions; hence through this book, we have tried to gather possible questions that can be presented as SBA. The book is divided into 11 chapters consisting of the questions from the 18 different modules covered in the examination. Questions are based on the themes of previous papers. Special features of this book are inclusion of the two Practice Question Papers (1 and 2) consisting of 50 questions each for practice. It provides the references for the answers given at the end of the chapter and covers the RCOG guidelines, not just the Green-top Guidelines, NICE Guidelines and the TOGs especially from last 3 years.

The book is designed to revise your factual knowledge as well as clinical application. While going through the questions, it is important to go through the references.

Each question is designed such that the important facts get ingrained in the brain. Considering the recent trend, *MRCOG Part-2* is presenting with lots of data and numbers in SBA questions, and we tried to present with questions on important data and numbers which is expected for the candidates to know.

The most productive way of using this book will be practice the questions on one topic and then go through the relevant guideline and research paper on the same topic. It will be very helpful to go through the book once again before exam, so that the numbers get ingrained in your brain.

The aim of MRCOG examination is to have a safe doctor with adequate evidence-based knowledge.

Special thanks to Dr Sridevi Vallabu (MBBS, MS, MRCOG), Registrar, Department of Obstetrics and Gynaecology at University Hospital of Coventry and Warwickshire NHS Trust, UK, for her contributions in framing the questions in Chapters 7 and 9.

We wish you the best of luck for the future.

Shailaja Rao Puppala
Sushama Gupta

Acknowledgements

I thank my family members Alekhya, Anirudh and Pradeep Mallisetty, who helped me in achieving success in MRCOG examination and supported me in writing this book. I am interested in guiding and supporting my colleagues in clearing this examination.

—**Shailaja Rao Puppala**

I thank my husband Arun and son Yash, who have helped me by supporting in all possible manner in completing this book and without them this would not have been possible.

—**Sushama Gupta**

Contents

1. Surgeries in Obstetrics and Gynaecology   1
2. Antenatal Care   15
3. Maternal Medicine   27
4. Management of Labour, Delivery and Postpartum Problems   41
5. Gynaecological Problems   48
6. Infertility   55
7. Family Planning and Sexual Reproductive Health   66
8. Early Pregnancy Care   83
9. Gynaeoncology   88
10. Urogynaecology   96
11. Miscellaneous Topics   105

Appendices

Practice Question Paper 1   *116*
Practice Question Paper 2   *128*

CHAPTER 1

Surgeries in Obstetrics and Gynaecology

1. Incidence of serious complications after abdominal hysterectomy:
   A. 4/100
   B. 2/100
   C. 6/100
   D. 8/100
   E. 10/100
2. Incidence of maternal death after caesarean section:
   A. 1/1,200
   B. 1/12,000
   C. 1/120,000
   D. 12/100,000
   E. 12/1,000,000
3. Decision to delivery interval for a category 2 caesarean section is:
   A. 45 minutes
   B. 30–75 minutes
   C. 45–60 minutes
   D. 60 minutes
   E. 60–90 minutes
4. Planned caesarean section compared to vaginal birth reduces the incidence of:
   A. Cardiac arrest
   B. Early postpartum haemorrhage (PPH)
   C. Secondary PPH
   D. Neonatal intensive care admission
   E. Caesarean hysterectomy
5. General anaesthesia for unplanned caesarean section should include the following measures to reduce aspiration:
   A. Preoxygenation
   B. Cricoid pressure
   C. Rapid sequence induction
   D. Lateral tilt 15 degrees
   E. Antacids
6. Early discharge after caesarean section can be offered:
   A. 48 hours
   B. 24 hours
   C. 12 hours
   D. 6 hours
   E. 72 hours

7. In laparoscopic surgery, the highest risk of vascular injury are for all of the following except:
   A. Young
   B. Thin
   C. Patients with severe anorexia
   D. Multiparous
   E. Multiple surgeries

8. Palmer's point entry is recommended in all except:
   A. Women with morbid obesity
   B. Women who are thin
   C. Previous pelvic surgery
   D. Splenomegaly
   E. Midline surgeries

9. Secondary ports must be inserted under direct vision perpendicular to the skin while maintaining the pneumoperitoneum at:
   A. 5–8 mmHg
   B. 15–18 mmHg
   C. 20–25 mmHg
   D. 15–20 mmHg
   E. 25–30 mmHg

10. Factors associated with uterine trauma at hysteroscopy include all except:
    A. Blind cervical dilatation
    B. Tortuous cervical canal
    C. Deviated uterine cavity
    D. Prostaglandin administration before surgery
    E. Inexperienced operator

11. Flexible hysteroscopes are associated with:
    A. Less pain during outpatient hysteroscopy
    B. Better images
    C. Fewer failed procedures
    D. Quicker examination time
    E. Reduced cost

12. Uterine distension with normal saline is better than in carbon dioxide in:
    A. Reducing the incidence of vasovagal episodes
    B. Improved image quality
    C. Procedure being performed quickly
    D. Less pain
    E. Used for operative vaginal delivery

13. There is a statistically significant difference in planned vaginal birth after caesarean (VBAC) and elective repeat caesarean section (ERCS):
    A. Thromboembolic disease
    B. Hysterectomy
    C. Endometritis
    D. Maternal death
    E. Depression

14. **Uterine rupture incidence with classical caesarean section:**
    A. 190/10,000
    B. 200-900/10,000
    C. 200/10,000
    D. 22-74/10,000
    E. 300/10,000
15. **Under enhanced recovery pathway dehydration is avoided by reducing the period of fluid fasting to:**
    A. 4 hours
    B. 2 hours
    C. 3 hours
    D. 6 hours
    E. 8 hours
16. **Intraoperative management under enhanced recovery includes:**
    A. Use of transverse incisions
    B. Epidural anaesthesia
    C. Use of nasogastric tube
    D. Individualized goal directed fluid therapy
    E. Minimally invasive surgery
17. **Which of the following tops the list of visceral damage related to laparoscopic pelvic surgery?**
    A. Bladder
    B. Bowel
    C. Ureter
    d. Common iliac
    E. Aorta
18. **The causes of inadvertent laparoscopic electrosurgical injuries are all except:**
    A. Inadvertent tissue contact
    B. Insulation failure
    C. Direct coupling
    D. Capacitive coupling
    E. Using brief intermittent activation
19. **Despite adequate precautions and repair of the bladder injury the incidence of fistula formation is:**
    A. 2%
    B. 5%
    C. 7%
    D. 9%
    E. 11%
20. **Surgical principles of ureteric repair are all except:**
    A. Water-tight and spatulated
    B. Tension free
    C. Absorbable and continuous sutures
    D. Avoid using too many sutures
    E. Use drainage
21. **Cerclage insertion is associated with an increase in:**
    A. Chorioamnionitis
    B. PPROM
    C. Induction of labour
    D. Maternal pyrexia
    E. Preterm labour

22. Women undergoing ultrasound indicated or rescue cerclage benefit from an inpatient stay of at least:
    A. 24 hours
    B. 24–48 hours
    C. 48 hours
    D. 48–72 hours
    E. 12–24 hours

23. All women with emergency caesarean section should receive thromboprophylaxis for at least:
    A. 7 days
    B. 10 days
    C. 3 days
    D. 5 days
    E. 14 days

24. Which suture is a monofilament, with good tensile strength and absorption of 90–120 days?
    A. Vicryl
    B. PDS
    C. Monocryl
    D. Maxon
    E. Catgut

25. This incision is used for caesarean section:
    A. Rocky-Davies
    B. Küstner
    C. Smead-Jones
    D. Jenkins
    E. McBurney incision

26. Most common site of uterine perforation is:
    A. Fundus
    B. Posterior wall
    C. Anterior wall
    D. Left lateral wall
    E. Right lateral wall

27. Antibiotics, observation and explanation to the patient are all that is usually necessary when a perforation occurs using all except:
    A. Resection loop
    B. During coil insertion
    C. Dilator
    D. Curette
    E. 5 mm hysteroscope

28. For disimpacting the head at full dilatation caesarean section the following have been described except:
    A. Whitmore position
    B. Silicone tube
    C. C-Snorkel
    D. Prague manoeuvre
    E. Patwardhan technique

29. In women with placenta praevia and previous caesarean section the incidence of emergency hysterectomy is:
    A. 27/100
    B. 21/100
    C. 23/100
    D. 11/100
    E. 18/100

30. Incidence of excessive bleeding requiring return to theatre after surgery for vaginal prolapse is:
    A. 2/100
    B. 4/100
    C. 7/1,000
    D. 9/1,000
    E. 11/1,000

31. **Regarding femoral neuropathy in gynaecology occur:**
    A. Excessive deep retractor blades
    B. Lateral placement of retractor
    C. Inappropriate lithotomy position
    D. Most common nerve injury
    E. Incidence is 7%

32. **Pes cavus deformity occurs due to injury to**
    A. Lateral cutaneous nerve
    B. Common peroneal nerve
    C. Tibial nerve
    D. Femoral nerve
    E. Genitofemoral

33. **Contraindications to suprapubic catheter use all excep**
    A. Very obese patient
    B. Severe pelvic trauma
    C. Suspicion of ovarian cyst
    D. Anticoagulation therapy
    E. Ascites

34. **Raising the catheter drainage bag above the bladder helps in dealing with:**
    A. Catheter bypass
    B. Catheter block
    C. Pain or discomfort
    D. Catheter balloon cuff formation or difficult removal
    E. Catheter balloon diffusion

35. **Limitations of laparoscopic treatment in adnexal cysts larger than 10 cm include**
    A. Spillage (chemical peritonitis, such as dermoid or unsuspected malignancy)
    B. Difficulty in introduction of Veress needle
    C. Limited visualisation of the ureter
    D. Technical challenge of retrieving the mass
    E. All of the above

ANSWERS

1. **(A) 4/100**

    Royal College of Obstetricians and Gynaecologists (RCOG): Consent Advice Number 4: Abdominal hysterectomy for benign conditions.

    The overall risk of serious complications from abdominal hysterectomy is approximately four women in every 100.

2. **(B) 1/12,000**

    RCOG: Consent Advice Number 7: Caesarean section.

    The serious maternal risks include death, approximately one woman in every 12,000 (very rare).

3. **(B) 30–75 minutes**

    NICE guideline on caesarean section:

    1.0.3 Decision-to-delivery interval for unplanned CS

    1.4.3.1 Perform category 1 and 2 CS as quickly as possible after making the decision, particularly for category 1 (new 2011)

    1.4.3.2 Perform category 2 CS in most situations within 75 minutes of making the decision (new 2011).

4. **(A) Cardiac arrest**

    NICE guideline caesarean section 1.1.2.1 Box A.

    Planned caesarean section compared with planned vaginal birth for women with an uncomplicated pregnancy and no previous caesarean section.

    Planned caesarean section may reduce the risk of the following in women:
    - Perineal and abdominal pain during birth and 3 days postpartum
    - Injury to vagina
    - Early postpartum haemorrhage
    - Obstetric shock.

    Planned caesarean section may increase the risk of the following in babies:
    - Neonatal intensive care unit admission.

    Planned caesarean section may increase the risk of the following in women:
    - Longer hospital stay
    - Hysterectomy caused by postpartum haemorrhage
    - Cardiac arrest.

5. **(D) Lateral tilt 15 degrees**

    NICE guideline caesarean section 1.4.5.8:

    General anaesthesia for unplanned CS should include preoxygenation, cricoid pressure and rapid sequence induction to reduce the risk of aspiration (2004, Amended 2011).

6. **(B) 24 hours**

   Length of hospital stay is likely to be longer after a CS (an average of 3–4 days) than after a vaginal birth (average 1–2 days). However, women who are recovering well, are apyrexial and do not have complications following CS should be offered early discharge (after 24 hours) from hospital and follow-up at home, because this is not associated with more infant or maternal readmissions (2004). NICE guideline caesarean section 1.6.7.1.

7. **(D) Multiparous**

   The Hasson technique or insertion at Palmer's point is recommended for the primary entry in women who are very thin, women at highest risk of vascular injury are the young, thin, nulliparous women with well-developed abdominal musculature; patients with severe anorexia are at particular risk. The aorta may lie less than 2.5 cm below the skin in these women RCOG Green-top Guidelines including British Society of Gynaecological Endoscopy (BSGE). Preventing entry-related gynaecological laparoscopic injuries, alternative sites of entry.

8. **(D) Splenomegaly**

   Palmer's point is the preferred alternative trocar insertion site, except in cases of previous surgery in this area or splenomegaly RCOG Green top Guidelines included in British Society of Gynaecological Endoscopy (BSGE). Preventing Entry-related Gynaecological Laparoscopic Injuries, alternative sites of entry.

9. **(C) 20–25 mmHg**

   RCOG Green-top Guidelines included in British Society of Gynaecological Endoscopy (BSGE). Preventing Entry-related Gynaecological Laparoscopic Injuries, Secondary ports.

10. **(D) Prostaglandin administration before surgery**

    RCOG Green-top Guideline number 59: Best Outpatient Practice in Hysteroscopy.

11. **(A) Less pain during outpatient hysteroscopy**

    Flexible hysteroscopes are associated with less pain during outpatient hysteroscopy compared with rigid hysteroscopes. However, rigid hysteroscopes may provide better images, fewer failed procedures, quicker examination time and reduced cost. Thus, there is insufficient evidence to recommend preferential use of rigid or flexible hysteroscopes for diagnostic outpatient procedures. Choice of hysteroscope should be left to the discretion of the operator. RCOG Green-top Guideline Number 59: Best Outpatient Practice in Hysteroscopy 7.2.

12. **(D) Less pain**

    For routine outpatient hysteroscopy, the choice of distension medium between carbon dioxide and normal saline should be left to the discretion of the operator as neither is superior in reducing pain, although uterine distension with normal saline appears to reduce the incidence of vasovagal episodes.

Uterine distension with normal saline allows improved image quality and allows outpatient diagnostic hysteroscopy to be completed more quickly compared with carbon dioxide.

Operative outpatient hysteroscopy, using bipolar electrosurgery, requires the use of normal saline to act as both the distension and conducting medium. RCOG Green-top Guideline Number 59: Best Outpatient Practice in Hysteroscopy.

8.1 Distension medium.

13. **(C) Endometritis**

    Royal College of Obstetricians and Gynaecologists (RCOG) Green-top Guideline Number 45: Birth after caesarea Section 6.3. Specific risks of vaginal birth after caesarean (VBAC) women undergoing planned VBAC compared with elective repeat caesarean section (ERCS) are at greater risk of blood transfusion requirement (170/10,000 vs 100/10,000) and endometritis (289/10,000 vs 180/10,000). There was no statistically significant difference between planned VBAC and ERCS groups in relation to hysterectomy (23/10,000 vs 30/10,000), thromboembolic disease (4/10,000 vs 6/10,000) or maternal death (17/100,000 vs 44/100,000).

14. **(B) 20—900/10,000**

    RCOG Green-top Guideline Number 45: Birth after caesarean section 6.2.

    Contraindications for VBAC: Due to higher absolute risks of uterine rupture or unknown risks, planned VBAC is contraindicated in women with previous uterine rupture—risk of recurrent rupture is unknown previous high vertical classical caesarean section (200–900/10,000 risk of uterine rupture) where the uterine incision has involved the whole length of the uterine corpus, three or more previous caesarean deliveries (reliable estimate of risks of rupture unknown).

15. **(B) 2 hours**

    Admission on the day of surgery has many advantage—these include reduction in preoperative bed usage. Dehydration is avoided by reducing the period of fluid fasting to 2 hours prior to anaesthetic, which has been shown to be safe without an increase the risk of aspiration. The use of complex carbohydrate drinks have been shown to be beneficial in colorectal surgery, reducing the length of stay and liked by patients. [Torbé, Crawford R, Nordin A, Acheson N. Enhanced recovery in gynaecology. The Obstetrician and Gynaecologist. 2013;15:26-8-(Perioperative care)].

16. **(C) Use of nasogastric tube**

    Enhanced recovery pathways advocate minimal access techniques. If considered necessary for the procedure to be performed safely, abdominal incisions should be as small as possible. Nasogastric, abdominal and vaginal drains have little benefit and should be avoided as they increase morbidity and prolong hospital stay. The routine use of vaginal packs has been questioned, not only because they are uncomfortable for patients but also because they may hinder, if not prevent, mobilisation. However, because of the lack of evidence, a departmental approach for their use should be adopted to ensure consistency. This is another area for research.

    Avoidance of intraoperative hypothermia has long been shown to reduce postoperative complications. In colorectal surgery, individualised goal-directed fluid therapy using stroke volume to guide intraoperative fluid management reduces peroperative mortality and length of stay. The benefit of this approach relates to a reduction in the risk of bowel hypoperfusion, but the role in gynaecological surgery is less clear. However, the use of intraoperative fluid management technologies is now recommended in patients undergoing major or high-risk surgery (including major surgery with an anticipated blood loss greater than 500 lL and major abdominal surgery) or high-risk patients (including patients aged over 80 years) undergoing intermediate-risk surgery. [Torbé E, Crawford R, Nordin A, Acheson N. Enhanced recovery in gynaecology. The Obstetrician and Gynaecologist. 2013;15:26–8. (Intraoperative care)]

17. **(A) Bladder**

    The urinary bladder is at risk of injury during laparoscopic gynaecological surgery, either due to the entry process (for example, during suprapubic port insertion) or due to its close association with the operating field (for example, during hysterectomy). In complex cases the bladder can also be at risk because of its direct involvement in the disease process (utero-vesical endometriotic nodule). The reported incidence varies greatly. Injury rates range from 0.02 to 8.3% placing bladder injury at the top of the list of visceral damage complications related to laparoscopic pelvic surgery. (Minas V, Gul N, Aust T, Doyle M, Rowlands D. Urinary tract injuries in laparoscopic gynaecological surgery; prevention, recognition and management. The Obstetrician and Gynaecologist. 2014 16:19-28.)

18. **(E) Using brief intermittent activation**

    Safety measures to prevent laparoscopic electrosurgical complications. Inspect insulation carefully before use. Use the lowest possible effective power setting. Use available technology; newer tissue response generators and active electrode monitoring technology eliminate concerns about insulation failure and capacitive coupling. Use a low-voltage waveform for monopolar diathermy (cut). Use bipolar electrosurgery when appropriate, use brief intermittent activation, do not activate in close proximity or direct contact with another instrument, ensure that both the heel and the tips of the bipolar forceps are kept under direct view when activating. (Minas V, Gul N, Aust T, Doyle M, Rowlands D. Urinary tract injuries in laparoscopic gynaecological surgery; prevention, recognition and management. The Obstetrician and Gynaecologist. 2014;16:1-28.)

19. **(B) 5%**

Bladder repairs should be watertight and leakage from the suture line should be tested (for example, with methylene blue or indigo carmine). A bladder catheter must be inserted and continuous postoperative bladder drainage should be allowed for 2 weeks. The above two measures (watertight closure and indwelling catheter) will improve healing and reduce the risk of subsequent vesicovaginal fistula formation. Prior to catheter removal, complete repair without leakage should be confirmed by retrograde cystography. If contrast escape is noted then the catheter should be left in situ and the test repeated in 1 week. Despite these measures, a fistula can still form with an approximate incidence of 5% (of the cases where an injury occurred). Even though management of these late presentations will usually be by open or vaginal route, several cases of successful laparoscopic repair of vesicovaginal fistulas have been reported to date. (Minas V, Gul N, Aust T, Doyle M, Rowlands D. Urinary tract injuries in laparoscopic gynaecological surgery; prevention, recognition and management. The Obstetrician and Gynaecologist. 2014;16:1-28).

20. **(C) Absorbable and continuous sutures**
    - Adequate but careful debridement to avoid shortening the ureter (debridement may be needed to enable the use of the healthy ureter for re-anastomosis)
    - Adequate but careful dissection to avoid devascularisation (dissection/mobilisation may be needed to lengthen the ureter for anastomosis)
    - Anastomosis must be:
        - Water-tight
        - Tension-free
        - Spatulated or fish-mouth
    - Use absorbable and intermittent sutures
    - Avoid using too many sutures
    - Use drainage (ureteral stents, bladder catheter, retr-peritoneal anastomotic site drain).

    Consider omental flap to cover the repair site and increase vascularity. When possible, repair by laparoscopy absorbable and intermittent sutures.

(Minas V, Gul N, Aust T, Doyle M, Rowlands D. Urinary tract injuries in laparoscopic gynaecological surgery; prevention, recognition and management. The Obstetrician and Gynaecologist. 2014;16:1-28).

21. **(D) Maternal pyrexi**

Although women are often routinely informed of a number of potential complications associated with cerclage insertion, including preterm premature rupture of membranes, miscarriage, preterm labour, infection, bleeding and bladder or cervical damage, there is little published evidence to support this. None of the randomised studies of cervical cerclage has been designed or adequately powered to assess the risk of maternal morbidity and, to date, none of the larger studies of history- or ultrasound-indicated cerclage has reported an increase in PPROM, preterm delivery or second-trimester loss.

Intraoperative complications including bladder damage, cervical trauma, membrane rupture and bleeding are reported but are rare (<1%).

An integrated project delivery (IPD) meta-analysis of seven randomised studies of cerclage insertion (combining data from studies of both history and ultrasound-indicated cerclage) found that cerclage was associated with an increased risk of maternal pyrexia ([odds ratio (OR) 2.35; 95% confidence interval (CI) 1.37–4.05)], but there was no evidence of increase in chorioamnionitis (OR 0.73; 95% CI 0.36–1.46), PPROM (OR 0.92; 95% CI 0.62–1.35), induction of labour or caesarean section (OR for spontaneous labour for no cerclage 0.81; 95% CI 0.65–1.02).

Royal College of Obstetricians and Gynaecologists Green-top Guideline Number 60: Cervical Cerclage.

What information should be given to the women regarding cerclage?

22. **(A) 24 hours**

Women undergoing ultrasound-indicated or rescue cerclage, given the higher risk of complications such as PPROM, early preterm delivery, miscarriage and infection, may benefit from at least a 24-hour postoperative period of observation in hospital. Cases should be managed on an individual basis.

In women undergoing insertion of transabdominal cerclage via laparotomy, an inpatient stay of at least 48 hours is recommended 24 hours RCOG Green-top Guideline Number 60: Cervical cerclage.

23. **(B) 10 days**

All women who have had caesarean sections should be considered for thromboprophylaxis with LMWH for 10 days after delivery apart from those having an elective caesarean section who should be considered for thromboprophylaxis with LMWH for 10 days after delivery if they have any additional risk factors.

RCOG Green-top Guideline Number Thrombosis and embolism during the pregnancy and puerperium, reducing the risk.

24. **(C) Monocryl**

    Raghavan R, Arya P, Arya P, China S. Abdominal incisions and sutures in obstetrics and gynaecology. The Obstetrician and Gynaecologist. 2014;16:1-18.

25. **(B) Küstner**

    The Küstner incision, sometimes incorrectly referred to as modified Pfannenstiel incision, involves a slightly curved skin incision beginning below the level of the anterior superior iliac spine and extending just below the pubic hairline. The superficial branches of the inferior epigastric artery or vein may be encountered in the fat. This incision is more time-consuming and extensibility is limited.

    Raghavan R, Arya P, Arya P, China S. Abdominal incisions and sutures in obstetrics and gynaecology. The Obstetrician and Gynaecologist. 2014;16:1-18.

26. **(C) Anterior wall**

    Early recognition and subsequent management will significantly reduce morbidity, long-term sequelae and possible mortality.

    Initially an injury can be suspected if extension of the instrument goes beyond the limitation of the uterus. Furthermore, loss of resistance with further instrumentation is highly indicative of a uterine perforation. Sudden loss of vision during hysteroscopic procedures due to collapse of the uterus and bleeding together with a large deficit of the distension medium is highly suggestive. Finally, direct visualisation of the perforation site, omentum or bowel is diagnostic. The site of perforation that is most common is the anterior wall of the uterus.

    Shakir F, Diab Y. The perforated uterus. The Obstetrician and Gynaecologist. 2013;15:25-61.

27. **(A) Resection loop**

    Management of uterine perforation will depend on the procedure being carried out and on the instruments used. If a perforation occurs when using a dilator, up to 5 mm hysteroscope, curette, during coil insertion, or polyp forceps, then antibiotics, observation and explanation to the patient is all that is necessary. If larger diameter instruments are used, tissues grasped and avulsion attempted, or if there is significant revealed bleeding from a uterine tear, then laparoscopy should be performed.

    Shakir F, Diab Y. The perforated uterus. The Obstetrician and Gynaecologist. 2013;15:25-61.

28. **(D) Prague manoeuvre**

    Patwardhan's method is described less commonly. This involves delivery of both fetal shoulders through the incision followed by the trunk, breech, and then finally lifting the head out of the pelvis. Optimal positioning of the woman, such as the Whitmore position (modified lithotomy where thighs are moderately abducted and flexed to 135° from the trunk), optimising the surgeon position, for example, use of a stool or low patient bed or use of non-dominant hand to apply an even traction to disimpact the head. The C-snorkel is an anatomically curved tube with multiple ventilation ports. It can be inserted between the vaginal wall and foetal head, and aeration through the ports can alleviate the vacuum between them, aiming to lessen the force required to disimpact the foetal head. The Foetal Disimpacting System® (Eurosurgical Ltd., Guildford, UK) consists of a silicone balloon that can be inserted through the vagina to rest under the foetal head. It can then be inflated with saline in an attempt to elevate the foetal head.

Vousden N, Cargill Z, Briley A, Tydema, G, Shennan AH. Caesarean section at full dilatation: incidence, impact and current management. The Obstetrician and Gynaecologist. 2014;16:19-205.

29. **(A) 27/100**

    RCOG Consent Advice Number 12: Caesarean section for placenta praevia.

30. **(A) 2/100**

    RCOG Consent Advice Number 5: Vaginal surgery for prolapse.

31. **(E) Incidence is 7%**

    Kuponiyi O, Alleemudder DI, Latunde-Dada A, Eedarapalli P. Nerve injuries associated with gynaecological surgery. The Obstetrician and Gynaecologist. 2014;16:2-36.

    Femoral neuropathy commonly occurs as a result of compression of the nerve against the pelvic sidewall as it emerges from the lateral border of the psoas muscle. This happens when excessively deep retractor blades are used or during the lateral placement of retractors. In a 10-year prospective study, Goldman et al. reported an 8% incidence of femoral neuropathy when self-retaining retractors were used during gynaecological surgery, compared to an incidence of <1% when not use. Inappropriate patient positioning in lithotomy is also another cause of stretch-related femoral neuropathy. Gynaecological surgery is the most common contributor to iatrogenic femoral nerve injury, and abdominal hysterectomy is mostly responsible for this. Of all reports of gynaecological associated neuropathy, the femoral nerve is most frequently implicated, with an incidence of at least 11%.

32. **(C) Tibial Nerve**

    Kuponiyi O, Alleemudder DI, Latunde-Dada A, Eedarapalli P. Nerve injuries associated with gynaecological surgery. The Obstetrician and Gynaecologist. 2014;16:2-36.

    Table 2 summary of lumbosacral plexus.

Tibial nerve supplies the toes, plantar surface of the foot and causes plantar flexion and inversion of the foot. Its injury causes pavus deformity of the foot.

33. **(B) Severe pelvic trauma**

    Aslam N, Moran PA. Catheter use in gynaecological practice. The Obstetrician and Gynaecologist. 2014;16:16-8.

    Contraindications
    - Absolute: Unexplained haematuria due to risk of placing the catheter through a bladder tumour.
    - Relative:
      - Extensive abdominal adhesions from previous surgeries, especially closed insertion
      - Extensive intraoperative bladder reconstruction
      - Anticoagulation therapy/blood clotting disorder
      - Inability to fill the bladder to a minimum of 300 mL
      - Ascites
      - Suspicion of ovarian cyst
      - Very obese patients.

34. **(C) Pain or discomfort**

    Aslam N, Moran PA. Catheter use in gynaecological practice. The Obstetrician and Gynaecologist. 2014;16:16-8.

    The eyelets of the catheter may be occluded by urothelium due to hydrostatic suction. Raise the drainage bag above the level of the bladder for 10–15 seconds, encourage mobilisation and fluid intake.

35. **(E) All of the above**

    Refer to Stavroulis A, Memtsa M, Yoong W. Methods for specimen removal from the peritoneal cavity after laparoscopic excision. The Obstetrician and Gynaecologist. 2013;15:2-30.

    Laparoscopy-assisted cystectomy for large adnexal cysts. Large adnexal cysts exceeding 10 cm on preoperative imaging can be initially decompressed either through ultrasound guided or laparoscopic aspiration followed by intracorporeal ovarian cyst wall stripping performed endoscopically. Limitations of laparoscopic treatment in these cases include spillage (chemical peritonitis, such as dermoid or unsuspected malignancy), difficulty in introduction Veress needle, limited visualisation of the ureters, and technical challenge of retrieving the mass.

CHAPTER 2

Antenatal Care

1. **What percentage of women goes into labour before a scheduled elective caesarean section?**
   A. 1%
   B. 5%
   C. 10%
   D. 20%
   E. 25%

2. **Best predictor for a successful vaginal birth after caesarean (VBAC) is:**
   A. VBAC at or after 41 weeks of gestation
   B. Previous vaginal birth
   C. Previous VBAC
   D. Cervical dilatation at admission less than 4 cm
   E. Previous CS for dystocia

3. **Contraindications for VBAC are following except:**
   A. Previous classical CS
   B. Previous uterine rupture
   C. Previous two caesarean section
   D. Previous high vertical classical CS
   E. None of the above

4. **Most consistent finding in uterine rupture is:**
   A. Vaginal bleeding
   B. Abnormal CTG
   C. Tenderness at scar site
   D. Loss of station
   E. Cessation of previous efficient uterine activity

5. **Risk of uterine rupture in unscarred uterus is:**
   A. 0.5–2/10,000
   B. 20/10,000
   C. 2–9/1,000
   D. 80/10,000
   E. 24/10,000.

6. **Monochorionic placenta can have to placental masses (bipartite) in:**
   A. 1% B. 3%
   C. 5% D. 10%
   E. 0.1%

7. **Diagnosis of TTS is based on following except:**
   A. Presence of two placental masses
   B. Concordant gender
   C. Discordant bladder appearance
   D. Oligohydramnios with MVP less than 2 cm in one sac and polyhydramnios in other sac
   E. Haemodynamic and cardiac compromise

8. **TTS may recur in:**
   A. 1% B. 3%
   C. 10% D. 14%
   E. 20%

9. **Risk of death of surviving twin after foetal death of the co-twin in a monochorionic pregnancy is:**
   A. 1% B. 5%
   C. 12% D. 18%
   E. 25%

10. **Most characteristic cause of perinatal loss in monoamniotic twin is:**
    A. TTS B. Discordant growth
    C. Cord entanglement D. TRAP
    E. Placental insufficiency

11. **Most common congenital heart defect in monoamniotic twin is:**
    A. Transposition of great arteries B. Fallot of tetralogy
    C. VSD D. Aortic stenosis
    E. PDA

12. **Antepartum haemorrhage complicates what percentage of pregnancies:**
    A. 1–2% B. 3–5%
    C. 5–7% D. 9–10%
    E. 12%

13. **Risk of abruption in a woman with previous two pregnancies complicated by abruption is:**
    A. 1–2% B. 4–5%
    C. 10–15% D. 20–25%
    E. 40%

14. **Risk factors for placenta praevia are following except:**
    A. Previous caesarean section B. Multiple pregnancy
    C. Smoking D. Assisted conception
    E. Raised BMI

15. A 25-year-old woman presents with vaginal bleed at 28 weeks of her third pregnancy. She is known rhesus-positive. The Keilhauer test shows FMH of 6 mL. How much anti-D should this woman receive?
    A. 250 IU
    B. 500 IU
    C. 625 IU
    D. 750 IU
    E. 1,000 IU

16. A primigravida opts for physiological third stage. After how long would you call it a prolonged third stage of labour?
    A. 20 minutes
    B. 30 minutes
    C. 45 minutes
    D. 60 minutes
    E. 90 minutes

17. Postnatal management of pregnancies complicated by major/massive haemorrhage with suboptimal outcome include following except:
    A. Good communication between maternity unit and women's GP/CMW
    B. Midwife led debriefing
    C. Clinical incident reporting
    D. Follow-up appointment in 4–6 weeks postnatal
    E. Debriefing

18. A 34-year-woman is in her fourth pregnancy; she had all her three pregnancies delivered by caesarean section. Her risk of placenta praevia is:
    A. 1:100
    B. 1:200
    C. 1:50
    D. 1:30
    E. 1:10.

19. Prophylactic oxytocic for management of third stage of labour can reduce PPH by up to:
    A. 10%
    B. 20%
    C. 40%
    D. 60%
    E. 75%

20. Therapeutic goals of management of massive blood loss is to maintain:
    A. Haemoglobin greater than 8 g/dL
    B. Prothrombin greater than 1.5 × mean control
    C. Activated prothrombin time less than 1.5 × mean control
    D. Fibrinogen greater than 1.0 g/L
    E. Platelets more than 75×10^9/L

21. A woman in her first pregnancy presents with PPROM at 32 weeks of gestation. She is tachycardia and febrile on admission. What proportions of PPROM are associated with intrauterine infections?
    A. 1%
    B. 10%
    C. 15%
    D. 25%
    E. 40%

22. **A woman at 28 weeks of gestation presents with malarial infection with confirmed *Plasmodium vivax*. The treatment of choice is:**
    A. Chloroquine
    B. Primaquine
    C. Quinine
    D. Quinine + Clindamycin
    E. Artesunate

23. **A nulliparous at 28 weeks gestation asks for advice regarding chemoprophylaxis against malaria as she is planning to travel to South Asia. What is the drug of choice for chemoprophylaxis?**
    A. Mefloquine
    B. Chloroquine
    C. Primaquine
    D. Proguanil
    E. None

24. **Highest incidence of obstetric cholestasis is seen in:**
    A. Indian
    B. Pakistani
    C. Araucanian-Indian
    D. Chile
    E. Caucasian

25. **Most reliable method of monitoring pregnancy complicated with obstetric cholestasis in order to predict foetal death is:**
    A. Ultrasound scan for growth
    B. CTG
    C. Biochemical monitoring of bile acid
    D. None
    E. All

26. **A 28-year-old nulliparous delivers a term stillbirth. What proportions of term stillbirths are associated with chromosomal abnormality?**
    A. 0.1%
    B. 1–2%
    C. 5–6%
    D. 10–12%
    E. 20%

27. **Optimal method of confirmation of intrauterine death (IUD) is:**
    A. Pinard stethoscope
    B. Doppler ultrasound
    C. Real time ultrasound
    D. Real-time ultrasound and colour Doppler
    E. MRI

28. **Risk of DIC after 4 weeks of IUD is:**
    A. 5%
    B. 10%
    C. 20%
    D. 30%
    E. 40%

29. **A woman develops malaria at 20 weeks of gestation. How should the baby be monitored post-delivery?**
    A. Thick and thin film at birth if normal discharge
    B. Thick and thin film weekly up till 28 days
    C. If placenta shows negative histopathology, discharge
    D. Observe for 72 hours
    E. Do nothing

30. **Periumbilical sparing is seen in following condition:**
    A. Atopic eruption of pregnancy
    B. Polymorphic eruption of pregnancy
    C. Pemphigoid gestationis
    D. Intrahepatic cholestasis
    E. All

31. **Following skin condition has an association with autoimmune condition:**
    A. Atopic eruption of pregnancy
    B. Polymorphic eruption of pregnancy
    C. Pemphigoid gestationis
    D. Intrahepatic cholestasis
    E. All

32. **Pemphigoid gestationis is associated with following except:**
    A. Autoimmune condition
    B. Appears around umbilicus as urticarial papule
    C. Sparing of palms and soles
    D. Postnatal flare up is common
    E. Newborn may develop self-limiting skin lesion

33. **The following are major risk factor for SGA except:**
    A. Maternal age more than 35 years
    B. Paternal SGA
    C. Renal impairment
    D. Heavy bleeding similar to menses
    E. PAPP-A less than 0.4 MoM

34. **A 35-year nulliparous presents to you in antenatal clinic, her BMI is 19. How would you manage her care?**
    A. Serial growth scans from 26 to 28 weeks
    B. Uterine artery Doppler at 20–24 weeks
    C. Commence low dose aspirin
    D. UAD at 20–24-week and serial growth scans from 26 to 28 weeks
    E. Do nothing

35. **In severe SGA, the incidence of chromosomal abnormalities can be up to:**
    A. 5%
    B. 12%
    C. 19%
    D. 30%
    E. 75%

36. **Autosomal dominant condition:**
    A. Dubin-Johnson
    B. Wilson's disease
    C. Fanconi's anaemia
    D. Gilbert syndrome
    E. Fabry's disease

37. **Advise pregnant women who have a sleep problem about sleep hygiene:**
    A. Healthy bedtime routine
    B. Avoiding caffeine
    C. Reducing activity before sleep
    D. Consider promethazine
    E. All the above

38. **High intensity psychological intervention therapy:**
    A. Depression, anxiety disorders, bipolar disorders
    B. Alcohol and drug misuse and sleep disorders
    C. Eating disorders
    D. A, B, C
    E. A, C

ANSWERS

1. **(C) 10%**

   As up to 10% of women scheduled for elective repeat caesarean section (ERCS) go into labour before the 39th week, it is good practice to have a plan for the event of labour starting prior to the scheduled date.
   Refer to Royal College of Obstetricians and Gynaecologists (RCOG) Green-top Guideline Number 45 (GTG Number 45).

2. **(C) Previous vaginal birth after caesarean (VBAC)**

   Previous vaginal birth, particularly previous VBAC, is the single best predictor for successful VBAC.
   Refer to RCOG (GTG Number 45).

3. **(C) Previous two caesarean section**

   Planned VBAC is contraindicated in women with:
   - Previous uterine rupture—risk of recurrent rupture is unknown
   - Previous high vertical classical caesarean section (200 the single best predictor for successful VB
     - The uterine incision has involved the whole length of the uterine corpus
     - Three or more previous caesarean deliveries (reliable estimate of risks of rupture unknown).

   Refer to RCOG (GTG Number 45).

4. **(B) Abnormal CTG**

   An abnormal cardiotocograph (CTG) is the most consistent finding in uterine rupture.
   Refer to RCOG (GTG Number 45).

5. **(A) 0.5–2/10,000**

   Uterine rupture in an unscarred uterus is extremely rare at 0.5 2.0/10,000 deliveries; this risk is mainly confined to multiparous women in labour.
   Refer to RCOG (GTG Number 45).

6. **(B) 3%**

   Three per cent of monochronic (MC) placentas have two placental masses (bipartite), so these are not necessarily dichorionic.
   Refer to RCOG (GTG Number 51).

7. **(B) Concordant gender**

   The diagnosis of twin-twin transfusion syndrome (TTTS) is based on ultrasound criteria:
   - The presence of a single placental mass
   - Oligohydramnios with maximum vertical pocket (MVP) less than 2 cm in one sac and polyhydramnios in other sac.

- Discordant bladder appearances—severe TTTS
- Haemodynamic and cardiac compromise—severe TTTS.

8. **(D) 14%**

   Twin-twin transfusion syndrome (TTTS) can recur later in up to 14% of pregnancies treated by laser ablation.

   Refer to RCOG (GTG Number 51).

9. **(C) 12%**

   After the single foetal death in a monochorionic pregnancy, the risk to the surviving twin of death or neurological abnormality is of the order of 12% and 18%, respectively.

   Refer to RCOG (GTG Number 51).

10. **(C) Cord entanglement**

    This is unique to monoamniotic twins and the incidence varies in published literature.

    Refer to The Obstetrician and Gynaecologist (TOG) 2012 Vol 14 Issue 2.

11. **(A) Transposition of great arteries**

    The incidence of congenital heart malformations is about 5% in monochorionic twins; some nine-fold higher than expected for singleton pregnancy. Transposition of the great arteries is the most common congenital heart defect in monoamniotic twins.

    Refer to TOG 2012 Vol 14 Issue 2.

12. **(B) 3–5%**

    APH complicates 3–5% of pregnancies and is a leading cause of perinatal morbidity and mortality. Up to one-fifth of very preterm babies are born in association with APH, and the known association of APH with cerebral palsy can be explained by preterm delivery.

    Refer to RCOG (GTG Number 63).

13. **(D) 20–25%**

    A large observational study from Norway reported a 4.4% incidence of recurrent abruption. Abruption recurs in 19% of women who have had two previous pregnancies complicated by abruption.

    Refer to RCOG (GTG Number 63).

14. **(E) Raised BMI**

    Risk factors for placenta praevia are listed in GTG Number 63.

    Refer to RCOG (GTG Number 63).

15. **(D) 750 IU**

    At least 500 IU anti-D should be administered intramuscularly (IM) and additional anti-D given if the FMH is confirmed to be more than 4 mL additional dose of anti-D immunoglobulin is necessary for larger FMH and the dose to be administered by intramuscular route should be calculated as 125 IU for each additional mL of FMH.

Antenatal Care

Refer to British Committee for Standards in Haematology (BCSH) guideline 2014.

16. **(C) 45 minutes**

    Diagnose a prolonged third stage of labour if it is not completed within 30 minutes of the birth with active management or within 60 minutes of the birth with physiological management.

    Refer to NICE Intrapartum care (December, 2014).

17. **(B) Midwife led debriefing**

    The postnatal management of pregnancies complicated by major or massive APH should include thromboprophylaxis, debriefing and clinical incident reporting. The events should be discussed and the woman and her family given the opportunity to ask questions. A follow-up appointment 4–6 weeks following birth should be offered and contact numbers for access to medical and psychological support should be provided as appropriate. The events should be discussed and the woman and her family given the opportunity to ask questions. A follow-up appointment 4–6 weeks following birth should be offered and contact numbers for access to medical and psychological support should be provided as appropriate.

    Refer to RCOG (GTG Number 63).

18. **(D) 1:30**

    Risk of placenta praevia in first pregnancy is 1:400, with 1 caesarean section is 1:160, with 2 caesarean section is 1:60, with 3 caesarean section is 1:30 and with 4 caesarean section is 1:10.

    Refer to RCOG (GTG Number 27).

19. **(D) 60%**

    Prophylactic oxytocic should be offered routinely in the management of the third stage of labour in all women as they reduce the risk of PPH by about 60%.

    Refer to RCOG (GTG Number 52).

20. **(B) Prothrombin greater than 1.5 × mean control**

    A 2006 guideline from the British Committee for Standards in Haematology summarises the main therapeutic goals of management of massive blood loss is to maintain:

    - Haemoglobin greater than 8 g/dL
    - Platelet count more than 75×10^9/L
    - Prothrombin less than 1.5 × mean control
    - Activated prothrombin times less than 1.5 × mean control
    - Fibrinogen greater than 1.0 g/L.

    Refer to RCOG (GTG Number 52).

21. **(C) 15%**

    Preterm premature rupture of membranes (PPROM) complicates only 2% of pregnancies but is associated with 40% of preterm deliveries and can result in significant neonatal morbidity and mortality. Women with intrauterine infection deliver earlier than non-infected women and infants born with sepsis have mortality four times higher than those without sepsis. Foetal tachycardia predicts 20–40% of cases of intrauterine infection with a false positive rate of about 3%.

    Refer to RCOG (GTG Number 44).

22. **(A) Chloroquine**

    Non-falciparum malaria like *Plasmodium vivax, Plasmodium ovale, Plasmodium malariae* are treated with oral chloroquine (base) 600 mg followed by 300 mg 68 hours later. Then 300 mg on day 2 and again on day 3.

    Refer to RCOG (GTG Number 54B).

23. **(A) Mefloquine**

    Mefloquine (5 mg/kg once a week) is the recommended drug of choice for prophylaxis in the second and third trimesters for chloroquine-resistant areas.

    Refer to RCOG (GTG Number 54A).

24. **(C) Araucanian-Indian**

    In England, obstetric cholestasis (also referred to as intrahepatic cholestasis of pregnancy) affects 0.7% of pregnancies in multi-ethnic populations 1 and 1.2 cholestasis (also referred to as intrahepatic cholestasis of pregnancy) affects 0.7% of pregnancies in multi-ethnic mortality birth with physiological management. For example, in Chile, 2.4% of all pregnancies are affected, with a 5% prevalence in women of Araucanian-Indian origin.

    Refer to RCOG (GTG Number 43).

25. **(D) None**

    Poor outcome cannot currently be predicted by biochemical results and delivery decisions should not be based on results alone.

    No specific method of antenatal foetal monitoring for the prediction of foetal death can be recommended.

    Ultrasound and cardiotocography are not reliable methods for preventing foetal death in obstetric cholestasis.

    Continuous foetal monitoring in labour should be offered.

    Refer to RCOG (GTG Number 43).

26. **(C) 5–6%**

    Karyotyping is important as about 6% of stillborn babies will have a chromosomal abnormality.

    Refer to RCOG (GTG Number 55).

27. **(D) Real-time ultrasound and colour Doppler**

    Real-time ultrasonography is essential for the accurate diagnosis of intrauterine foetal death (IUFD).

    Ideally, real-time ultrasonography should be available at all times.

    A second opinion should be obtained whenever practically possible. Real-time ultrasound allows direct visualization of the foetal heart. Imaging can be technically difficult, particularly in the presence of maternal obesity, abdominal scars and oligohydramnios, but views can often be augmented with colour Doppler of the foetal heart and umbilical cord.

    Refer to RCOG (GTG Number 55).

28. **(D) 30%**

    There is also a moderate risk of maternal disseminated intravascular coagulation (DIC): 10% within 4 weeks after the date of late IUFD, rising to 30% thereafter.

    Refer to RCOG (GTG Number 55).

29. **(B) Thick and thin film weekly up till 28 days**

    All neonates whose mothers developed malaria in pregnancy should be screened for malaria with standard microscopy of thick and thin blood films at birth and weekly blood films for 28 days.

    Refer to RCOG (GTG Number 54B).

30. **(B) Polymorphic eruption of pregnancy.**

    The condition initially presents with pruritic, erythematous papules commonly located within the abdominal striae and with periumbilical sparing. It progresses to the trunk and extremities, sparing the palms and soles in the majority of cases, and does not affect the face. The condition initially presents with pruritic, erythematous papules commonly located within the abdominal striae and with periumbilical sparing. It progresses to the trunk and extremities, sparing the palms and soles in the majority of cases, and does not affect the face.

    Refer to TOG Vol 15 No 4 2013.

31. **(A) Atopic eruption of pregnancy**

    The incidence of this dermatosis is very rare, affecting between 1 in 1,700 and 1 in 50,000 pregnancies. There is a recognised correlation with the haplotypes HLA-DR3 and HLA-DR4.

    Refer to TOG Vol 15 No 4 2013.

32. **(C) Sparing of palms and soles**

    The rash usually appears around the umbilicus as urticarial papules and plaques, which join to form bullae, extending to involve the trunk, extremities, palms and soles with mucosal sparing. Large, tense blisters can form after a few weeks around the edge of the rash or in otherwise unaffected areas of the skin.

    Refer to TOG Vol 15 No 4 2013.

33. **(A) Maternal age more than 35 years**

    List of major risk factors for small for gestational age (SGA) are age more than 40, maternal and paternal SGA, smokes more than 10 cigarettes, cocaine, daily vigorous exercise, previous SGA and stillbirth, chronic hypertension, diabetes with vascular disease, renal impairment, anti-phospholipid syndrome, heavy bleeding similar to menses, PAPP-A less than 0.4 MoM.

    Refer to RCOG (GTG Number 31).

34. **(B) Uterine artery Doppler at 20–24 weeks**

    Women who have three or more minor risk factors should be referred for uterine artery Doppler at 20% areas of the skin.

    Refer to RCOG (GTG Number 31).

35. **(C) 19%**

    In severe SGA, the incidence of chromosomal abnormalities has been reported to be as high as 19%. Triploidy was the most common chromosomal defect in foetuses referred before 26 weeks of gestation and trisomy 18 in those referred thereafter.

    Refer to RCOG (GTG Number 31).

36. **(D) Gilbert syndrome**

    Gilbert's syndrome is a common genetic liver disorder found in 3–12% of population. There is elevated levels of unconjugated bilirubin, normally has no serious consequences, although mild jaundice may appear under conditions of stress. There is reduction in the glucuronidation activity of the enzyme, (UGT1A1).

    Refer to Genetic Home Reference. February 2012.

37. **(E) All the above**

    Interventions for sleep problems

    1.8.21 Antenatal and postnatal mental health: clinical management and service guidance (CG192).

38. **(E) A, C**

    Antenatal and postnatal mental health: clinical management and service guidance (CG192).

CHAPTER 3

Maternal Medicine

1. According to UK Immunisation Schedule in Pregnancy ideally the pertussis vaccine should be offered to pregnant women:
   A. After first trimester
   B. In third trimester
   C. After third trimester
   D. 28–38 weeks
   E. 28–32 weeks.

2. Vaccines recommended in pregnancy in certain situations:
   A. Hepatitis A vaccine, rabies vaccine, typhoid vaccine
   B. Meningococcus vaccine, hepatitis B vaccine
   C. Yellow fever vaccine
   D. A and B
   E. All the above

3. With a proven primary infection of toxoplasmosis the risk of having an affected foetus is highest:
   A. Less than 12 weeks
   B. 12–20 weeks
   C. 13–28 weeks
   D. 20–28 weeks
   E. More than 36 weeks.

4. Incidence of gestational diabetes in women:
   A. 87.5%
   B. 75.5%
   C. 67.5%
   D. 82.7%
   E. 77.5%

5. Pregnant women are advised with any form of diabetes to maintain their fasting capillary plasma glucose below the target levels of:
   A. 5.5 mmol/L
   B. 5.3 mmol/L
   C. 5.7 mmol/L
   D. 5.1 mmol/L
   E. 6.0 mmol/L

6. Advise women with uncomplicated gestational diabetes to give birth by:
   A. 38 + 6 weeks
   B. 39 + 6 weeks
   C. 37 + 6 weeks
   D. 40 + 6 weeks
   E. 41 weeks

7. Offer a trial of changes in diet and exercise to women with gestational diabetes who have a fasting plasma glucose level?
   A. Below 7 mmol/L at diagnosis
   B. Below 8 mmol/L at diagnosis
   C. Below 6.5 mmol/L at diagnosis
   D. Below 7.5 mmol/L at diagnosis
   E. Below 5.7 mmol/L at diagnosis

8. Which drug can be considered for women with gestational diabetes in whom blood glucose targets are not achieved with metformin but who decline insulin therapy or who cannot tolerate metformin?
   A. Glibenclamide   B. Glicazide
   C. Acarbose   D. Glipizide
   E. Pioglitazone

9. In pre-eclampsia how many term babies are small for gestational age (SGA):
   A. 5–10%   B. 10–15%
   C. 15–20%   D. 20–25%
   E. 17–23%

10. Recurrence of gestational hypertension in future pregnancy is:
    A. 1/6   B. 1/10
    C. 1/15   D. 1/20
    E. 1/25

11. In pregnant women with target organ damage secondary to chronic hypertension the aim is to keep the blood pressure less than:
    A. 150/100   B. 140/100
    C. 150/90   D. 140/90
    E. 135/100

12. The following is a complication of severe eclampsia:
    A. Hypernatraemia
    B. Hyponatraemia
    C. Hypokalaemia
    D. Hyperkalaemia
    E. Hypermagnesaemia

13. Magnesium sulphate is used in the management of pre-eclampsia in all the following except:
    A. Abnormal liver enzymes alanine aminotransferase (ALT) or aspartate aminotransferase (AST) above 70
    B. Platelet count below 150
    C. Papilloedema
    D. Clonus more than three beats
    E. Liver tenderness

14. **Ultrasound assessment of foetal growth and liquor volume and Doppler is done twice in all the following are except:**
    A. Previous pre-eclampsia with SGA
    B. Previous intrauterine death
    C. Previous abruption
    D. Previous pre-eclampsia with birth less than 37 weeks
    E. Previous severe pre-eclampsia
15. **Cardiotocography is indicated in the following conditions except:**
    A. Chronic hypertension
    B. Severe gestational hypertension with abdominal pain
    C. Mild pre-eclampsia with bleeding
    D. Weekly in pre-eclampsia
    E. Diagnosis of severe gestational hypertension
16. **If the women has taken methyldopa for treatment of hypertension it should be stopped within how many days:**
    A. 2 days   B. 5 days
    C. 7 days   D. 10 days
    E. 2 weeks
17. **Prevalence of asthma in pregnancy is:**
    A. 3–7%   B. 5–9%
    C. 4–12%   D. 10–15%
    E. 20%
18. **Exacerbation is are most common in asthma at:**
    A. Less than 12 weeks   B. 12–24 weeks
    C. 24–36 weeks   D. 36–40 weeks
    E. No change with gestation
19. **Which prostaglandin is not associated with bronchospasm?**
    A. Prostaglandin F2α   B. Prostaglandin E2
    C. Prostaglandin E1   D. Syntometrine
    E. All of the above
20. **Congenital heart block in systemic lupus erythematosus has a recurrence rate of**
    A. 5%   B. 8%
    C. 10%   D. 16%
    E. 18%
21. **The following help in differentiating lupus nephritis from pre-eclampsia except:**
    A. Fall in complement
    B. Presence of haematuria
    C. Presence of red cell casts
    D. Presence of proteinuria
    E. Renal biopsy

22. **Antiphospholipid antibodies (APA) are present in systemic lupus erythematosus (SLE) in about:**
    A. 15% of women
    B. 20% of women
    C. 25% of women
    D. 30% of women
    E. 35% of women

23. **Drug-induced lupus is caused by:**
    A. Quinidine
    B. Cyclophosphamide
    C. Methotrexate
    D. Dexamethasone
    E. Azathioprine

24. **Hypothyroidism in pregnancy leads to the following complications:**
    A. Anaemia
    B. Placental abruption
    C. Postpartum haemorrhage
    D. Pre-eclampsia
    E. Depression

25. **How many cases of hypothyroidism are missed with only high-risk screening?**
    A. 1/4
    B. 1/5
    C. 1/3
    D. 1/2
    E. 1/7

26. **In hypothyroidism thyroid stimulating hormone (TSH) level should be maintained at:**
    A. Below .5 mU/L
    B. Below 2.5 mU/L
    C. Above 2.5 mU/L
    D. Below 3 mU/L
    E. Above 3 mU/L

27. **Chlamydia in a 28-week pregnant women is treated by:**
    A. Azithromycin 1 g PO with no test of cure if asymptomatic
    B. Azithromycin 1 g PO test of cure in 6 weeks
    C. Azithromycin 1 g PO test of cure in 5 weeks
    D. Amoxicillin 500 mg TDS for 5 days
    E. Erythromycin 250 mg QDS for 2 weeks

28. **Regarding anogenital warts in pregnancy:**
    A. There is no vertical transmission
    B. There is vertical transmission and treatment reduces the risk of vertical transmission
    C. Vertical transmission occurs in 1/200 and treatment reduces the risk of vertical transmission
    D. Vertical transmission occurs in 1/80 and treatment reduces the risk of vertical transmission
    E. Vertical transmission occurs 1/80 and the treatment does not reduce the risk

29. **Chronic complications of sickle cell disease:**
    A. Pulmonary hypertension
    B. Nephropathy
    C. Proliferative retinopathy
    D. Iron deficiency anaemia
    E. Intrauterine growth restriction

30. The second most common organism causing urinary tract infection (UTI) in pregnancy:
    A. *Escherichia coli*
    B. *Proteus mirabilis*
    C. *Staphylococcus saprophyticus*
    D. *Klebsiella*
    E. *Mixed anaerobes*

31. Pregnancy appears to have a minimal adverse effect on the long-term graft prognosis, provided that pre-pregnancy renal function is satisfactory that is:
    A. Serum creatinine less than 125 μmol/L
    B. Serum creatinine less than 140 μmol/L
    C. Serum creatinine less than 130 μmol/L
    D. Serum urea less than 95 μmol/L
    E. Serum urea of less than 80 μmol/L

32. Magnetic resonance imaging (MRI) improves the diagnosis and alters counselling in all except:
    A. Corpus callosum abnormalities
    B. Cortical dysplasia
    C. Cytomegalovirus infection
    D. Complex multisystem disorders
    E. Foetal hydrops

33. Most common central nervous system (CNS) anomalies diagnosed and missed by ultrasound:
    A. Ventriculomegaly and agenesis of corpus callosum
    B. Holoprosencephaly and ventriculomegaly
    C. Agenesis of cerebellum vermis and agenesis of corpus callosum
    D. Meningomyelocele and ventriculomegaly
    E. Agenesis of corpus callosum and holoprosencephaly

34. MRI has a limited role in the following conditions except:
    A. Assessment of the surviving twin in monochorionic twins
    B. Genitourinary abnormalities
    C. Vascular lesions in the brain
    D. Site and size of the congenital diaphragmatic hernia
    E. Assessment of abdominal cavity

35. Regarding Zika virus transmission which statement is not true:
    A. It is transmitted only through mosquito bite
    B. If a female partner is pregnant, condom use is advised for a male traveller to reduce the risk of transmission during travel
    C. If a female partner is at risk of getting pregnant from effective contraception is advised to prevent pregnancy and condom use is advised for a male traveller to reduce the risk of transmission during travel

D. If a female partner is at risk of getting pregnant from effective contraception is advised to prevent pregnancy and condom use is advised for a male traveller for 28 days after his return from an active Zika transmission area if he has not had any symptoms compatible with Zika virus infection
E. If a female partner is at risk of getting pregnant, or is planning pregnancy, effective contraception is advised to prevent pregnancy and condom use is advised for a male traveller for 1 year following the start of symptoms if a clinical illness compatible with Zika virus infection or laboratory confirmed Zika virus infection was reported.

Maternal Medicine

ANSWERS

1. **(E) 28–32 weeks**

   Pregnant women should be offered the diphtheria, tetanus, pertussis (whooping cough) and polio (DTaP/IPV) vaccine in 28–38 weeks of their pregnancy (ideally in 28–32 weeks), for each pregnancy. The pertussis vaccine can be given at the same time as the influenza vaccine but pertussis vaccination should not be given early in order to offer the vaccines at the same time as this will compromise the passive protection to the infant.

2. **(D) Hepatitis A vaccine, Hepatitis B vaccine, Rabies vaccine, Typhoid vaccine, Meningococcal vaccine**

   Vaccines recommended in pregnancy in certain situations
   - Hepatitis A vaccine, hepatitis B vaccine, meningococcus vaccine, pneumococcal vaccine
   - Rabies vaccine
   - Typhoid vaccine
   - Yellow fever vaccine.

   Arunakumari PS, Kalburgi S, Sahare A. Vaccination in pregnancy. The Obstetrician and Gynaecologist. 2015;17:257-63.

3. **(C) 13–28 weeks**

   Foetal transmission risk increases with gestational age at seroconversion (from <1% before 4 weeks, between 4% and 15% at 13 weeks, to >60% at 36 weeks). Conversely, the risk of congenital abnormality is inversely related to the gestation at maternal infection, such that the severity is greatest when infection occurs during the first trimester. Thus, the combined risk of having an affected foetus, given proven maternal primary infection, is highest in the middle of pregnancy, at 13–28 weeks.

   To M, Kidd M, Maxwell D. Prenatal diagnosis and management of fetal infections. The Obstetrician and Gynaecologist. 2009;11:108-116. doi: 10.1576/toag.11.2.108.27484.

4. **(A) 87.5%**

   Of women who have diabetes during pregnancy, it is estimated that approximately 87.5% have gestational diabetes (which may or may not resolve after pregnancy), 7.5% have type 1 diabetes and the remaining 5% have type 2 diabetes.

5. **(B) 5.3 mmol/L**

   Advise pregnant women with any form of diabetes to maintain their capillary plasma glucose below the following target levels, if these are achievable without causing problematic hypoglycaemia. Fasting: 5.3 mmol/L. 1.3.5.

6. **(D) 40 + 6 weeks**

   Advise women with uncomplicated gestational diabetes to give birth no later than 40 + 6 weeks.

7. **(A) Below 7 mmol/L at diagnosis**

   Offer a trial of changes in diet and exercise to women with gestational diabetes who have a fasting plasma glucose level below 7 mmol/L at diagnosis. 1.2.23.

8. **(A) Glibenclamide**

   Consider glibenclamide for women with gestational diabetes:

   In whom blood glucose targets are not achieved with metformin but who decline insulin therapy or who cannot tolerate metformin.

9. **(D) 20–25%**

   Small for gestational age babies (mainly because of foetal growth restriction arising from placental disease) are common, with 20–25% of preterm births and 14–19% of term births in women with pre-eclampsia being less than the tenth centile of birth weight for gestation. [NICE clinical guideline (CG107)].

10. **(A) 1/6**

    Tell women who had gestational hypertension that their risk of developing: gestational hypertension in a future pregnancy ranges from about 1 in 6 (16%) pregnancies to about 1 in 2 (47%) pregnancies. [NICE Guidance CG107 (1.10.4.1)].

11. **(D) 140/90**

    1.2.3.3 Offer pregnant women with target-organ damage secondary to chronic hypertension (for example, kidney disease) treatment with the aim of keeping blood pressure lower than 140/90 mmHg. NICE Guidance CG107.

12. **(D) Hyperkalaemia**

    1.8.7.1 Complications:
    - Eclampsia
    - HELLP syndrome
    - Haemorrhage
    - Hyperkalaemia
    - Severe oliguria
    - Coagulation support
    - Intravenous antihypertensive treatment
    - Initial stabilisation of severe hypertension
    - Evidence of cardiac failure
    - Abnormal neurology.

13. **(B) Platelet count below 150**

    1.8.1.3 Mild or moderate hypertension and proteinuria with one or more of the following:
    - Symptoms of severe headache
    - Problems with vision, such as blurring or flashing before the eyes
    - Severe pain just below the ribs or vomiting
    - Papilloedema
    - Signs of clonus (≥3 beats)
    - Liver tenderness
    - HELLP syndrome
    - Platelet count falling to below $100 \times 10^9/L$
    - Abnormal liver enzymes [alanine aminotransferase (ALT) or aspartate aminotransferase (AST) rising to above 70 IU/L].

14. **(D) Previous pre-eclampsia with birth less than 37 weeks**

    1.6.4.1 Carry out ultrasound foetal growth and amniotic fluid volume assessment and umbilical artery Doppler velocimetry starting at between 28 weeks and 30 weeks (or at least 2 weeks before previous gestational age of onset if earlier than 28 weeks) and repeating 4 weeks later in women with previous:
    - Severe pre-eclampsia
    - Pre-eclampsia that needed birth before 34 weeks
    - Pre-eclampsia with a baby whose birth weight was less than the 10th centile
    - Intrauterine death
    - Placental abruption.

15. **(A) Chronic hypertension**

    1.6.1.2 In women with chronic hypertension, only carry out cardiotocography if foetal activity is abnormal.

16. **(A) 2 days**

    1.5.3.6 If a woman has taken methyldopa to treat pre-eclampsia, stop within 2 days of birth.

17. **(C) 4–12%**

    The prevalence of asthma in pregnant women is 4–12%, making it the most common chronic condition in pregnancy. Pregnancy can affect asthma control and conversely asthma can affect pregnancy.

18. **(C) 24–36 weeks**

    In severe disease, asthma control is more likely to deteriorate (~60%) than in mild disease (~10%). Exacerbations are most common between 24 weeks and 36 weeks of pregnancy. Respiratory viral infections were the most frequent triggers of exacerbations (34%), followed by poor adherence to inhaled corticosteroid therapy (29%). Therefore, during pregnancy women with asthma need to be closely reviewed throughout pregnancy, irrespective of disease severity.

19. **(A) Prostaglandin F2α**

    Prostaglandin F2α (for example, Hemabate®, Pfizer Ltd., Sandwich, UK) can cause bronchospasm and needs to be used with caution, whereas prostaglandin E2 (for example, Prostin®, Pharmacia Ltd, Sandwich, UK) is not associated with bronchospasm. Asthma in Pregnancy TOG September 2013.

20. **(D) 16%**

    The usual presentation is a fixed foetal bradycardia of 60–80 beats per minute on ultrasound scan. It occurs in 2–3% of foetuses of women with the anti-Ro/La antibody and there is a recurrence rate of 16% in subsequent pregnancies. It is associated with significant perinatal morbidity and mortality, with about half of infants requiring pacing by the first year of life. Congenital heart block develops between 18–28 weeks of gestation and foetal echocardiography should be performed around this period to detect it. Hydrops faetalis can occur in utero and is thought to be due to the degree of endomyocardial fibrosis and associated myocarditis.

21. **(B) Presence of haematuria**

    The features of lupus nephritis include hypertension and proteinuria with or without haematuria and renal impairment. Lupus nephritis is caused by autoantibodies which produce immune complexes: these are deposited in the kidneys and they activate the complement cascade, causing a generalised inflammatory response. The presence of haematuria or red cell casts as well as a rise in anti-dsDNA titres or a fall in complement levels help to distinguish this from pre-eclampsia; in addition, lupus disease activity in non-renal organ systems suggests that a lupus nephritis flare is more likely. New-onset lupus nephritis without a previous history of renal involvement is unusual but not impossible.

    Despite these distinguishing features the only definitive and reliable investigation that can be used to distinguish pre-eclampsia from lupus nephritis is renal biopsy.

22. **(D) 30% of women**

    Antiphospholipid antibodies are present in about 30% of women with SLE and are associated with arterial and venous thrombosis, recurrent miscarriage, foetal growth restriction, foetal loss and preterm delivery due to utero-placental insufficiency; they require specific management.

23. **(D) Dexamethasone**

    The most common of these are hydralazine, procainamide, quinidine, isoniazid, diltiazem and minocycline. The pathophysiology of drug-induced lupus is not completely understood, but in the case of hydralazine, it is thought to be caused by the formation of antinuclear antibodies to H1 and the H3–H4 complex (anti-histone). However, these drugs do not cause disease flare in women with established lupus.

Cauldwell M, Nelson-Piercy C. Maternal and fetal complications of systemic lupus erythematosus. The Obstetrician and Gynaecologist. 2012;14:167-174.

24. **(E) Depression**

    Complications of hypothyroidism include—anaemia, placental abruption, postpartum haemorrhage, cardiac dysfunction and pre-eclampsia.

    Jefferys A, Vanderpump M, Yasmin E. Thyroid dysfunction and reproductive health. The Obstetrician and Gynaecologist. 2015;17:39-45.

25. **(C) 1/3**

    History of thyroid dysfunction/thyroid surgery, family history of thyroid disease.
    - Goitre
    - Positive thyroid autoantibodies.

    Clinical symptoms/signs of hypothyroidism diabetes type I
    - History of miscarriage/preterm delivery
    - Other autoimmune disorders.

    History of subfertility
    - History of therapeutic head or neck irradiation
    - Age more than or equal to 30 years
    - Previous treatment with amiodarone
    - Previous treatment with lithium
    - Recent exposure to iodinated radiological contrast agents.

    As targeted screening of high-risk cases has been found to miss approximately one-third of cases of overt and subclinical hypothyroidism. At present a high-risk screening approach is currently adopted, therefore women at high risk should be screened.

    Jefferys A, Vanderpump M, Yasmin E. Thyroid dysfunction and reproductive health. The Obstetrician and Gynaecologist. 2015;17:39-45.

26. **(B) Below 2.5 mU/L**

    Given that improvements in reproductive outcomes are seen in those in whom the serum thyroid-stimulating hormone (TSH) is less than 2.5 mU/L, serum TSH levels should be maintained below 2.5 mU/L for those with both clinical and subclinical hypothyroidism. A first finding of subclinical hypothyroidism (serum TSH of more than 2.5 mU/L with normal free T4) should prompt a repeat serum TSH level and for thyroid autoantibodies to be checked. If the serum TSH persists above 2.5 mU/L, treatment with L-T4 is warranted to bring the TSH below 2.5 mU/L. The dose of L-T4 should be titrated until the serum TSH is brought to 2.5 mU/L or less, and during this period monitoring of LT4-4 and TSH every 6 weeks is warranted. The evidence is lacking over the benefit of commencing L-T4 in those who are euthyroid with autoimmune thyroid disease (AITD). It should, however, prompt close monitoring of thyroid function if pregnancy and monitoring of foetal well-being and subsequently neonatal review.

Jefferys A, Vanderpump M, Yasmin E. Thyroid dysfunction and reproductive health. The Obstetrician and Gynaecologist. 2015;17:39-45.

1.5.3.13 If biochemical and haematological indices are improving but stay within the abnormal range in women with pre-eclampsia who have given birth, repeat platelet count, transaminases and serum creatinine measurements as clinically indicated and at the postnatal review (6–8 weeks after the birth).

1.5.2.7 Recommend birth within 24–48 hours for women who have pre-eclampsia with mild or moderate hypertension after 37 + 0 weeks.

Recommend birth for women who have pre-eclampsia with severe hypertension after 34 weeks when their blood pressure has been controlled and a course of corticosteroids has been completed (if appropriate).

In women with mild hypertension presenting before 32 weeks, or at high risk of pre-eclampsia (see 1.1.1.1), measure blood pressure and test urine twice weekly.

Small for gestational age babies (mainly because of foetal growth restriction arising from placental disease) are common, with 20–25% of preterm births and 14–19% of term births in women with pre-eclampsia being less than the tenth centile of birth weight for gestation.

27. **(B) Azithromycin 1 g PO test of cure in 6 weeks**

    Table 1 Screening tests, sites, indications and recommended treatment and follow-up of sexually transmitted infections (STIs) in pregnancy.

    Allstaff S, Wilson J. The management of sexually transmitted infections in pregnancy. The Obstetrician and Gynaecologist. 2012;14:25-32.

    Women who have chlamydia treated in pregnancy are at increased risk of a positive subsequent test because of treatment failure or re-infection, hence the importance of public health interventions. A test of cure should be performed 5–6 weeks after completion of treatment and repeat screening in the third trimester is recommended.

28. **(D) Vertical transmission occurs in 1/80 and treatment reduces the risk of vertical transmission**

    Vertical transmission of human papillomavirus (HPV) occurs in up to 1 in 80 cases and can cause genital and laryngeal warts in infants. A rare complication of vertical transmission of low-risk.

    Human papillomavirus subtypes are recurrent respiratory papillomatosis, which occur in approximately 4.3 out of 1,00,000 cases. Although caesarean section has been shown to reduce the risk of this complication, it is rare compared with the frequency of maternal HPV infection, so operative delivery would not normally be advised. Treatment of anogenital warts in pregnancy does not reduce the risk of vertical transmission, so no treatment is an option.

Allstaff S, Wilson J. The management of sexually transmitted infections in pregnancy. The Obstetrician and Gynaecologist. 2012;14:25-32.

29. **(D) Iron deficiency anaemia.**

Screening for iron overload. In women who have been multiply transfused in the past or who have a high ferritin level, T2* cardiac magnetic resonance imaging may be helpful to assess body iron loading. Aggressive iron chelation before conception is advisable in women who are significantly iron loaded.

Green top guideline 61. Management of Sickle cell disease in pregnancy.

30. **(C)** *Staphylococcus saprophyticus*.

UTI in pregnancy TOG 2008.

Escherichia coli accounts for 80–90% of infections but other gram-negative bacilli, such as *Proteus mirabilis* and *Klebsiella pneumoniae*, can be cultured. *Proteus, Klebsiella* and most *Enterobacteriaceae* species show urease activity and form urinary calculi, which can act as reservoirs of infection. The coagulase negative cocci, *Staphylococcus saprophyticus*, is the second most frequently cultured uropathogen, while other gram-positive cocci, such as group B haemolytic streptococci, are less frequently isolated but remain clinically important.

31. **(A) Serum creatinine less than 125 μmol/L**

TOG Chronic renal disease complicating pregnancy July 2009.

The following guidelines have been recommended for women who have had renal transplants who are contemplating pregnancy
- There should have been no rejection in the previous year
- Graft function should be adequate and stable
- There should be no or minimal proteinuria (<500 mg/24 hours).

32. **(E) Foetal hydrops**

Magnetic resonance imaging (MRI) may improve diagnosis and alter counselling and projected prognosis for many lesions, such as corpus callosum abnormalities and cortical dysplasia. Overall comparing ultrasound and MRI diagnoses in foetuses with suspected CNS abnormalities, MRI altered the diagnosis in 32% of cases and counselling altered in approximately 50% of cases. Other studies have revealed that additional information could be obtained using MRI for conditions such as cytomegalovirus infection (abnormal gyration cerebellar hypoplasia or white matter abnormalities) and complex multisystem disorders.

---

*STIR weighted MRI images.

Story L, Rutherford M. Advances and applications in foetal magnetic resonance imaging. The Obstetrician and Gynaecologist. 2015.

33. **(A) Ventriculomegaly and agenesis of corpus callosum**

    Story L, Rutherford M. Advances and applications in fetal magnetic resonance imaging. The Obstetrician and Gynaecologist. 2015.

34. **(E) Assessment of abdominal cavity**

    Story L, Rutherford M. Advances and applications in fetal magnetic resonance imaging. The Obstetrician and Gynaecologist. 2015.

35. **(E) If a female partner is at risk of getting pregnant, or is planning pregnancy, effective contraception is advised to prevent pregnancy and condom use is advised for a male traveller for 1 year following the start of symptoms if a clinical illness compatible with Zika virus infection or laboratory confirmed Zika virus infection was reported.**

    Women whose partner has been to an area with Zika virus transmission

    As discussed above, almost all cases of Zika virus infection are acquired via mosquito bites. A small number of cases of sexual transmission of Zika virus have been reported, and in a limited number of cases, the virus has been shown to be present in semen, although it is not yet known how long this can persist. The risk of sexual transmission of Zika virus is thought to be low, but the number of reports is increasing.

    If a female partner is pregnant, condom use is advised for a male traveller to reduce the risk of transmission during travel and for the duration of the pregnancy.

    If a female partner is at risk of getting pregnant, or is planning pregnancy, effective contraception is advised to prevent pregnancy and condom use is advised for a male traveller to reduce the risk of transmission during travel and:
    - For 28 days after his return from an active Zika transmission area if he has not had any symptoms compatible with Zika virus infection
    - For 6 months following the start of symptoms if a clinical illness compatible with Zika virus infection or laboratory confirmed Zika virus infection was reported.

    This is a precaution and may be revised as more information becomes available.

    Zika virus RNA has been detected in semen at two months following onset of typical acute Zika virus illness in a single case. The suggested 6 months period of condom use for men who had suspected or confirmed Zika virus infection reflects a precautionary approach whilst further evidence is gathered. Refer to Zika virus infection RCOG website.

CHAPTER 4
Management of Labour, Delivery and Postpartum Problems

1. **Planned caesarean section may increase the risk of the following in women:**
   A. Longer hospital stay, hysterectomy caused by postpartum haemorrhage (PPH) and early PPH
   B. Cardiac arrest, longer hospital stay and hysterectomy caused by postpartum haemorrhage and early PPH
   C. Perineal and vaginal pain, cardiac arrest and PPH
   D. Injury to vagina, PPH and longer hospital stay
   E. Obstetric shock, PPH and perineal and abdominal pain on Day 3

2. **Foetal fibronectin testing is considered positive if concentration is more than:**
   A. 200 ng/mL
   B. 150 ng/mL
   C. 100 ng/mL
   D. 50 ng/mL
   E. Any amount irrespective of the value

3. **From 42 weeks women who decline induction of labour should be offered monitoring:**
   A. Alternate day cardiotocography (CTG) and Doppler
   B. Twice weekly CTG and weekly Doppler
   C. Twice weekly CTG and amniotic fluid measurement
   D. Twice weekly CTG, Amniotic fluid measurement with Doppler
   E. Alternate day CTG and twice weekly amniotic fluid measurement with Doppler

4. **Significant hyperbilirubinemia is more likely in all the babies except:**
   A. Gestational age under 38 weeks
   B. A previous sibling with neonatal jaundice requiring phototherapy
   C. Mother's intention to breastfeed exclusively
   D. Instrumental delivery
   E. Visible jaundice in the first 24 hours of life

5. **Vacuum extraction compared with forceps is no more likely to be associated with:**
   A. Cephalhaematoma, retinal haemorrhages and maternal worries about the baby
   B. Phototherapy, cephalhaematoma, delivery by caesarean section
   C. Delivery by caesarean section, phototherapy, retinal haemorrhages
   D. Low 5-minute Apgar score, delivery by caesarean section, phototherapy
   E. Maternal worries about the baby, phototherapy and delivery by caesarean section

6. **Women presenting with signs and symptoms of acute pulmonary embolism (PE) should have the following investigations to diagnose initially:**
   A. Arterial blood gas (ABG) and ECG
   B. ABG, ECG and chest X-ray
   C. ECG and chest X-ray
   D. Compression duplex ultrasound with chest X-ray
   E. All of the above

7. **Which tests should be performed routinely in case of a late intrauterine device (IUD):**
   A. Routine biochemistry with C-reactive protein (CRP) and bile salts
   B. Kleihauer test, occult maternal diabetes or thyroid
   C. Foetal and placental infections and occult maternal—foetal infections
   D. A and B
   E. A, B and C

8. **Women who have caesarean section:**
   A. Urinary tract infection (UTI), urge and stress incontinence
   B. UTI, urinary tract injury and stress incontinence
   C. Stress and urge incontinence, retention and urinary tract injury
   D. UTI, retention of urine and urinary tract injury
   E. All of the above

9. **Risk factors for obstetric anal sphincter injuries are:**
   A. Advanced maternal age, multipara, shoulder dystocia
   B. Nulliparous, Asian ethnicity, prolonged second stage
   C. Occipitoposterior position, birthweight more than 4 kg
   D. A and C
   E. B and C

10. **In shoulder dystocia the success rate of McRoberts manoeuvre alone is:**
    A. 80%
    B. 85%
    C. 90%
    D. 75%
    E. 70%

Management of Labour, Delivery and Postpartum Problems

11. **When should women be assessed about the resolution of symptoms of baby blues and evaluated further if needed?**
    A. 6 weeks postpartum
    B. 4 weeks postpartum
    C. 1 week postpartum
    D. 10–14 days postpartum
    E. All the time

12. **Indicators of successful breastfeeding are:**
    A. Relaxed arms and hands, breast softening, compression of nipple at the end of the feed
    B. Moist mouth, women feel content and active, breast softening
    C. Visible swallowing, moist mouth, compression of nipple at the end of the feed
    D. Less areola visible underneath the chin than above the nipple, sustained rhythmic suck, women feel relaxed and sleepy
    E. Vigorous cry, pink extremities and weight gain

13. **Regarding obstetric antenatal thromboprophylaxis risk assessment which of the following is correct:**
    A. 3 or more risk factors start from 12 weeks
    B. 4 or more risk factors start from 28 weeks
    C. 2 or more risk factors start from 36 weeks
    D. 3 or more risk factors start from 28 weeks and 4 or more from 12 weeks
    E. 2 or more risk factors start from 28 weeks and 3 or more from 12 weeks

14. **The following is not an indication (red flag sign) urgent referral for hospital assessment in puerperium:**
    A. Tachypnoea
    B. Anxiousness
    C. Offensive vaginal discharge
    D. Diarrhoea and/or vomiting
    E. Abdominal pain

15. **Non-steroidal anti-inflammatory drugs (NSAIDs) should be avoided for pain relief in sepsis as:**
    A. They can increase the bleeding
    B. They might interact with the antibiotics
    C. They mask the signs of sepsis
    D. They interfere with the ability of polymorphs to fight against GAS infection
    E. They are addictive

16. **Epidural adverse effects is:**
    A. Pruritus and shivering
    B. Drowsiness and dizziness
    C. Neonatal convulsions
    D. Reduced respiratory rate
    E. Nausea and vomiting

17. **Mortality rate due to anaphylaxis is:**
    A. 1/1,000
    B. 1/10,000
    C. 2/10,000
    D. 1/1,000
    E. 5/1,000

ANSWERS

1. **(B) Cardiac arrest, longer hospital stay and hysterectomy caused by postpartum haemorrhage and early PPH**

   NICE CG132 Box A

   Planned caesarean section may increase the risk of the following in women:

   Longer hospital stay, hysterectomy caused by postpartum haemorrhage, cardiac arrest.

2. **(D) 50 ng/mL**

   Refer to NICE guideline 25—1.7.5.

3. **(C) Twice weekly CTG and amniotic fluid measurement**

   NICE guideline 1.2.1.4: From 42 weeks, women who decline induction of labour should be offered increased antenatal monitoring consisting of at least twice-weekly, cardiotocography and ultrasound estimation of maximum amniotic pool depth.

4. **(D) Instrumental delivery**

   NICE guideline CG98 1.2.1.

   Identify babies as being more likely to develop significant hyperbilirubinaemia if they have any of the following factors:
   - Gestational age under 38 weeks
   - A previous sibling with neonatal jaundice requiring phototherapy
   - Mother's intention to breastfeed exclusively
   - Visible jaundice in the first 24 hours of life.

5. **(C) Delivery by caesarean section, phototherapy, retinal haemorrhages**

   Refer to RCOG Green-top Guideline Number 26—Operative Vaginal Delivery:

   Vacuum extraction compared with forceps is more likely to fail delivery with the selected instrument, cephalhaematoma, retinal haemorrhage, maternal worries about baby.

   It is less likely to be associated with significant maternal perineal and vaginal trauma and no more likely to be associated with delivery by caesarean section, low 5-minute Apgar score or the need for phototherapy.

6. **(C) ECG and chest X-ray**

   Refer to Green-top Guideline Number 37. 4.2 In pregnancy and the puerperium, one study found that the ECG was abnormal in 41% of women with acute PE; the most common abnormalities were T wave inversion (21%), $S_1Q_3T_3$ pattern (15%) and right bundle branch block (18% during pregnancy and 4.2% in the puerperium). Given the increasing incidence of ischaemic heart disease in pregnancy, the ECG may also be helpful in identifying alternative diagnoses. In the same cohort of women, ABG analysis showed that only 10% had arterial PO_2 levels less than 60 mmHg and 2.9% had oxygen saturation levels less than 90%. These findings indicate a diagnostic role for ECG in women with suspected acute PE, and that ABG analysis is of limited diagnostic value.

Chest X-ray (CXR) may identify other pulmonary disease such as pneumonia, pneumothorax or lobar collapse. While the CXR is normal in over half of pregnant patients with objectively proven PE, abnormal features caused by PE include atelectasis, effusion, focal opacities, regional oligaemia or pulmonary oedema. The radiation dose to the foetus from a CXR performed at any stage of pregnancy is negligible (less than 0.01 mSv). A CXR should be performed before deciding upon further diagnostic tests.

7. **(E) A, B and C**
   Green-top Guideline Number 55 (Table 1).

8. **(B) UTI, urinary tract injury and stress incontinence**
   NICE guideline CG132 1.7.1.4.
   Healthcare professionals caring for women who have had a caesarean section and who have urinary symptoms should consider the possible diagnoses of urinary tract infection, stress incontinence (occurs in about 4% of women after caesarean section), Urinary tract injury (occurs in about 1/1,000 caesarean section).

9. **(E) B and C**
   Green-top-Guideline No 29. 5.1.

10. **(C) 90%**
    Green-top-Guideline No 42: 6.3.1 How should shoulder dystocia be managed?

11. **(D) 10–14 days postpartum**
    NICE guideline 37—Postnatal care:
    1.2.25 At 10–14 days after birth, women should be asked about resolution of symptoms of baby blues (for example, tearfulness, feelings of anxiety and low mood). If symptoms have not resolved, the woman should be assessed for postnatal depression, and if symptoms persist, evaluated further (urgent action).

12. **(D) Less areola visible underneath the chin than above the nipple, sustained rhythmic suck, women feel relaxed and sleepy**
    NICE guideline 37—1.3.21 BOX 1.
    Postnatal care
    - Indicators of good attachment and positioning:
      - Mouth wide open, less areola visible underneath the chin than above the nipple

- Chin touching the breast, lower lip rolled down and nose free, no pain
- Indicators of successful feeding in babies:
  - Audible and visible swallowing, sustained rhythmic suck, relaxed arms and hands, moist mouth
  - Regular soaked/heavy nappies
- Indicators of successful breastfeeding in women:
  - Breast softening, no compression of the nipple at the end of the feed, woman feels relaxed and sleepy.

13. **(D) 3 or more risk factors start from 28 weeks and 4 or more from 12 weeks**

    Refer to Reducing the Risk of Venous Thromboembolism during Pregnancy and the Puerperium. Green-top Guideline Number 37 Appendix 1.

14. **(C) Offensive vaginal discharge**

    Refer to Green-top Guideline Number 64b: Bacterial Sepsis Following Pregnancy.

    Red flag' signs and symptoms (see below) should prompt urgent referral for hospital assessment and, if the woman appears seriously unwell, by emergency ambulance:
    - Pyrexia more than 38°C
    - Sustained tachycardia more than 90 beats/minute
    - Breathlessness (respiratory rate >20 breaths/minute; a serious symptom) abdominal or chest pain
    - Diarrhoea and/or vomiting
    - Uterine or renal angle pain and tenderness.

    Woman is generally unwell or seems unduly anxious or distressed.

15. **(D) They interfere with the ability of polymorphs to fight against GAS infection**

    Refer to Green-top Guideline Number 64b—Bacterial Sepsis Following Pregnancy.

    Non-steroidal anti-inflammatory drugs (NSAIDs) should be avoided for pain relief in cases of sepsis as they impede the ability of polymorphs to fight GAS infection.

16. **(A) Pruritus and shivering**

    Refer to Alleemudder DI, Kuponiyi Y, Kuponiyi C, McGlennan A, Fountain S, Kasivisvanathan R. Analgesia for labour: an evidence-based insight for the obstetrician. The Obstetrician and Gynaecologist. 2015;17:147.

    Epidural side effects
    - Failure to work (1 in 10)
    - Pruritus and shivering

- Significant hypotension (1 in 50)
- Severe headache (1 in 100)
- Temporary nerve damage (1 in 1,000)
- Permanent nerve damage (1 in 13,000)
- Infection, meningitis, epidural blood clot (<1 in 50,000).

17. **(D) 1/1,000**

    Refer to Green-top Guideline Number 56—Maternal Collapse in Pregnancy and Puerperium. 4.2.9 Anaphylaxis.

CHAPTER 5

Gynaecological Problems

1. **The level of testosterone to prompt for the investigation of causes other than polycystic ovary syndrome (PCOS) is:**
   A. Less than 2 nmol/L
   B. 2–5 nmol/L
   C. More than 5 nmol/L
   D. More than 7 nmol/L
   E. More than 15 nmol/L

2. **Anorexia nervosa:**
   A. A higher incidence of hyperemesis gravidarum
   B. A higher incidence of foetal abnormality
   C. Significantly high caesarean section rate
   D. Development of children born is affected
   E. Mother and baby bonding has been shown to be a problem

3. **Obesity:**
   A. Reduces bone density
   B. Increase in fibroids
   C. Delays menopause
   D. Decreases the vasomotor symptoms of menopause
   E. Poorer sexual functioning

4. **Premature ovarian failure incidence:**
   A. 1% in less than 40 years and ovarian activity resumes in 5–10%
   B. 1% in more than 40 years and ovarian activity resumes in 10–15%
   C. 1% in less than 40 years and ovarian activity resumes in 5–10%
   D. A definite cause is identified in 20–30%
   E. 1% in less than 40 years and 1% in more than 40 years

5. **Uterine arteriovenous malformations are associated with all except:**
   A. Infections
   B. Gestational trophoblastic disease
   C. Intrauterine contraception
   D. Pelvic trauma
   E. Gynaecological malignancies

6. In the management of menstrual problems in adolescent girls with learning and physical difficulties the combined oral contraceptive pill has the following advantages:
   A. No interaction with enzyme inhibiting drugs
   B. Low BMI so less risk of deep vein thrombosis (DVT)
   C. No interaction with enzyme inducing drugs
   D. Compliance will not be a problem
   E. Useful for girls with gastric feeding tubes requiring long-term enteral nutrition

7. McCune Albright syndrome is treated by:
   A. Glucocorticoids with mineralocorticoids
   B. Anastrozole
   C. Selective oestrogen receptor modulators—tamoxifen
   D. Hydrocortisone
   E. Selective serotonin uptake inhibitors

8. Central precocious puberty is associated with:
   A. Raised oestradiol levels
   B. Prolactinaemia
   C. Uterine volume of more than 5 mL
   D. Bone age diminished by 3 years
   E. Luteinising hormone (LH)/follicle-stimulating hormone (FSH) more than 1

9. Core or typical premenstrual disorder is diagnosed by all the following except:
   A. Symptoms being are not well defined
   B. Symptoms causing distress and impairment of daily life
   C. There is no relation with ovulation
   D. There is a symptom-free week between menstruation and ovulation
   E. There is no underlying physical disorder

10. Hysteroscopic resection of endometrial polyps is superior to blind avulsion techniques due to all of the following except:
    A. Reduced recurrence of polyps
    B. Uterine perforation risk reduction
    C. False passage risk reduction
    D. Less chances of missing the malignant cells at the base
    E. Cannot be done as outpatient without cervical dilatation

11. Postmenopausal bleeding is caused by endometrial carcinoma in:
    A. 2–5%
    B. 10%
    C. 15%
    D. 20%
    E. 25%

12. **Most common complication of uterine artery embolisation is:**
    A. Severe pain
    B. Precipitate menopause
    C. Expulsion of necrotic fibroids
    D. Infection
    E. Vaginal discharge

13. **Pelvic congestion syndrome is definitely diagnosed by:**
    A. History and clinical features
    B. CT/MRI
    C. Venography
    D. Laparoscopy
    E. Ultrasound

ANSWERS

1. **(C) More than 5 nmol/L**

   Many practitioners believe that a serum total testosterone of less than 5.0 nmol/L, measured using an extraction immunoassay, makes serious pathology in a female unlikely. Mild hyperandrogenism with a serum total testosterone level of around 2-5 nmol/L is thought to be consistent with PCOS, while marked elevations (>5 nmol/L) should prompt investigation for other causes, such as an androgen secreting tumour. Refer to TOG July, 2013.

2. **(D) Development of children born is affected**

   Refer to TOG July, 2012—Anorexia nervosa in pregnancy.

   The children tended to weigh less and their weight correlated inversely with the mother's concern about her own body shape. However, the only long-term study 32 to date (a Danish prospective cohort followed up to 12.5 years) showed no difference in the development of the children born to mothers with anorexia nervosa compared with those from the general population.

3. **(D) Decreases the vasomotor symptoms of menopause**

   Perimenopausal women commonly seek medical attention for relief of vasomotor symptoms associated with menopause. Hot flushes have been shown to have an effect on sleep, quality of life and mood. The incidence of these symptoms has also been shown to increase in those with obesity. Metabolic syndrome, which is known to be associated with obesity, has also been identified to be associated with poorer sexual functioning.

   Refer to TOG July, 2015: Impact of obesity in the health of women in midlife.

4. **(A) 1% in less than 40 years and ovarian activity resumes in 5-10%**

   Diagnosis and management of premature ovarian failure. Refer to TOG, 2011.

5. **(C) Intrauterine contraception**

   Acquired arteriovenous malformations (AVMs) are also associated with infection, inflammation, retained products of conception, gestational trophoblastic disease, gynaecologic malignancies, pelvic trauma and exposure to Diethylstilboestrol. They have however, also been described in adolescent girls and postmenopausal women.

6. **(E) Useful for girls with gastric feeding tubes requiring long-term enteral nutrition**

   According to the Society for Adolescent Health and Medicine (SAHM) clinical guidelines 21 for treating adolescents who do well on DMPA for contraception, the physicians should continue prescribing DMPA to adolescent girls needing contraception, while providing adequate explanation of benefits and potential risks, consider ordering a DXA scan to evaluate a patient's risk; keep in mind that duration of use need not be restricted to 2 years, recommend 1,300 mg calcium plus 400 IU vitamin D and daily exercise to all adolescents receiving DMPA, consider oestrogen supplementation in those girls with osteopenia (or those at high risk of osteopenia who have not had a DXA scan) who are otherwise doing well on DMPA and have no contraindication to oestrogen.

The World Health Organization (WHO) similarly published recommendations stating that no restriction should be placed on the use of DMPA due to bone effects. A further practical issue that must be addressed is the weight gain associated with the DMPA (up to 4.6 kg/year). This additional weight may severely impact on quality of life, particularly if the girls are immobile and represents a major concern for parents or carers if they have to be lifted.

7. **(B) Anastrozole**

Suppression of gonadal steroidogenesis with aromatase inhibitors (which inhibit synthesis of oestrogen): first (testolactone), second and third-generation (anastrozole and letrozole) available. Treatment of peripheral precocious puberty.

Tirumuru SS, Arya P, Latthe P. Understanding precocious puberty in girls. The Obstetrician and Gynaecologist. 2012;14:121-9.

8. **(E) Luteinising hormone (LH)/follicle-stimulating hormone (FSH) more than 1**

The bone age is advanced, often by more than 2 years. A uterine volume more than 2 mL or length more than 34 mm, a pear-shaped uterus and endometrial thickening (endometrial echo) on pelvic ultrasound are associated with progressive central precocious puberty (CPP). Baseline serum gonadotrophins may be raised. The gonadotropin-releasing hormone (GnRH) luteinising hormone-releasing hormone (LHRH) stimulation test is the gold standard test for diagnosing CPP. It is performed by measuring follicle-stimulating hormone (FSH) and luteinising hormone (LH) levels sequentially after administering a GnRH analogue bolus. In healthy pubertal children, the LH response exceeds the FSH response. In pre-pubertal children and in thelarche variant, the FSH response exceeds the LH response. In cases of CPP, GnRH stimulation shows a pubertal response with luteinising hormone predominance (LH:FSH ratio >1). Peak LH levels vary, depending on the specific assay used, but values of more than 8 IU/L are usually considered diagnostic of CPP.

Tirumuru SS, Arya P, Latthe P. Understanding precocious puberty in girls. The Obstetrician and Gynaecologist. 2012;14:121.

9. **(C) There is no relation with ovulation**

   Criteria for diagnosing core premenstrual disorder are:
   - It is precipitated by ovulation
   - Symptoms are not defined, although typical symptoms exist
   - Any number of symptoms can be present
   - Physical and psychological symptoms are important
   - Symptoms recur in the luteal phase symptoms disappear by the end of menstruation
   - A symptom-free week occurs between menstruation and ovulation
   - Symptoms must be prospectively rated
   - Symptoms are not an exacerbation of an underlying psychological or physical disorder
   - Symptoms cause significant distress and impairment of daily activities, such as work commitments, social interactions and family activities.

   Walsh S, Ismaili E, Naheed B, O'Brien S. Diagnosis, pathophysiology and management of premenstrual syndrome. The Obstetrician and Gynaecologist. 2015;17:99-104.

10. **(E) Cannot be done as outpatient without cervical dilatation**

    There is good direct and circumstantial evidence that hysteroscopic resection of endometrial polyps under vision is safe, simple and superior to blind techniques:

    Malignant cells at the base of the polyp can be missed with blind avulsion. Hysteroscopic resection avoids excessive cervical dilatation which is when uterine perforation and creation of a false passage usually occur. Not a single recurrence of endometrial polyps was reported when resection under vision was compared with removal with a grasping forceps (recurrence rate 15%).

    Annan JJ, Aquilina J, Ball E. The management of endometrial polyps in the 21st century. The Obstetrician and Gynaecologist. 2012;14:33-8.

11. **(B) 10%**

    Pathological findings in patients with postmenopausal bleeding.

    Otify M, Fuller J, Ross J, Shaikh H, Johns J. Endometrial pathology in the postmenopausal woman—an evidence based approach to management. The Obstetrician and Gynaecologist. 2015;17:29-38.

12. **(E) Vaginal discharge**

    The Royal College of Obstetricians and Gynaecologists and the Royal College of Radiologists.

    Clinical recommendations on the use of uterine artery embolisation (UAE) in the management of fibroids, Third edition. London: RCOG and RCR, 2013.

13. **(C) Venography**

Venography remains the definitive imaging modality used to evaluate patients with pelvic congestion syndrome. The presence of one or more of the following venographic appearances is said to be suggestive of PCS:
- Ovarian vein diameter more than 10 mm
- Uterine venous engorgement
- Congestion of the ovarian plexus
- Filling of the pelvic veins across the midline and/or filling of the vulvovaginal thigh varicosities.

Osman MW, Nikolopoulos I, Jayaprakasan K, Raine-Fenning N. Pelvic congestion syndrome. The Obstetrician and Gynaecologist. 2013;15;151-7.

CHAPTER 6

Infertility

1. Infertility affects how many heterosexual couples in UK?
   A. 1/8
   B. 1/5
   C. 1/7
   D. 1/9
   E. 1/3

2. World Health Organization (WHO) reference value for the normal forms of spermatozoa in a semen analysis is:
   A. 15%
   B. 11%
   C. 7%
   D. 4%
   E. 9%

3. An earlier referral for specialist consultation to discuss the options for attempting conception, further assessment and appropriate treatment should be offered to:
   A. Woman is aged 35 years or over
   B. Woman is aged 36 years or over
   C. Man aged 40 years or over
   D. Woman more than 35 years and man more than 45 years
   E. Single women

4. The following does not improve the chances of pregnancy in endometriosis IUI:
   A. Surgical ablation in mild/minimal endometriosis
   B. Surgical ablation in moderate/severe endometriosis
   C. Ovarian cystectomy
   D. Postoperative medical management
   E. Intrauterine insemination (IUI)

5. In vitro fertilisation (IVF) treatment should be offered in unexplained infertility after:
   A. 2 years of unprotected sexual intercourse
   B. 2 years of fertility investigations
   C. 1 year of unprotected sexual intercourse
   D. After intrauterine insemination
   E. 1 year of unprotected sexual intercourse and fertility investigations

6. **Unstimulated intrauterine insemination can be considered in all except:**
   A. People who are unable to, have vaginal intercourse
   B. People who would find it very difficult to, have vaginal intercourse
   C. Are using partner or donor sperm
   D. People with unexplained infertility
   E. People in same-sex relationships

7. **When using gonadotrophins for ovarian stimulation in IVF cycle, use an individualised starting dose of follicle-stimulating hormone (FSH), based on factors that predict success, such as:**
   A. Age
   B. BMI
   C. Past history of ovarian hyperstimulation syndrome (OHSS)
   D. Ovarian reserve
   E. Presence of polycystic ovaries

8. **Replacement of embryos is into a uterine cavity is not recommended when the endometrium is:**
   A. Less than 5 mm
   B. Less than 3 mm
   C. More than 7 mm
   D. Less than 7 mm
   E. More than 3 mm

9. **Maximum dosage of FSH per day in for ovarian stimulation in IVF:**
   A. 500 IU
   B. 750 IU
   C. 450 IU
   D. 250IU
   E. 600 IU

10. **The preferred cryopreservation technique for sperm is:**
    A. Freezing in liquid nitrogen
    B. Freezing in carbon dioxide
    C. Vitrification
    D. Hatching
    E. Freezing in dry ice

11. **Cryopreserved material is stored for an initial period of:**
    A. 25 years
    B. 10 years
    C. 7 years
    D. Lifetime
    E. 14 years

12. **Mild forms of OHSS in in vitro fertilisation cycle are common, incidence being:**
    A. Up to 33%
    B. Up to 13%
    C. 3–8%
    D. 13–18%
    E. 20-25%

13. **Differential diagnosis for ovarian hyperstimulation syndrome are all except:**
    A. Ovarian cyst (torsion, haemorrhage)
    B. Pelvic infection
    C. Ectopic pregnancy
    D. Irritable bowel syndrome
    E. Appendicitis

14. **Hypoproteinaemia is a criteria for the diagnosis of:**
    A. Moderate OHSS
    B. Severe OHSS
    C. Critical OHSS
    D. Major OHSS
    E. None of the above

15. **The Human Fertilisation and Embryology Authority (HFEA) Standards for Assisted Conception Centres states that all adverse incidents occurring at the treatment centre for OHSS must be reported by telephone to the HFEA within:**
    A. 12 working hours of the identification of the incident and submission of an Incident Report Form within 24 working hours
    B. 24 working hours of the identification of the incident and submission of an Incident Report Form within 12 working hours
    C. 24 working hours of the identification of the incident and submission of an Incident Report Form within 48 working hours
    D. 48 working hours of the identification of the incident and submission of an Incident Report Form within 24 working hours
    E. 12 working hours of the identification of the incident and submission of an Incident Report Form within 48 working hours

16. **Women at higher risk of developing OHSS are:**
    A. Polycystic ovaries
    B. Under 30 years of age
    C. Use of GnRH antagonists
    D. Exposure to LH
    E. Exposure to HCG

17. **Electrolyte imbalance seen in OHSS is:**
    A. Hyperkalaemia and hypocalcaemia
    B. Hypokalaemia and hypernatraemia
    C. Hypernatraemia and hypokalaemia
    D. Hyponatraemia and hyperkalaemia
    E. Hypocalcaemia and hypokalaemia and hyponatraemia

18. **Intra-abdominal pressure of greater than how much is suggestive of decompression in OHSS:**
    A. 25 mmHg
    B. 20 mmHg
    C. 18 mmHg
    D. 15 mmHg
    E. 10 mmHg.

19. **Thrombosis incidence, site and system involved in OHSS are**
    A. 7–10%, upper body, arterial system
    B. 5–3%, upper body, arterial system
    C. 7–10%, upper body, venous system
    D. 5–3%, lower body, venous system
    E. 5–10%, lower body, venous system

20. **Pre-testicular causes of male infertility due to hypogonadotrophic hypogonadism accounts for:**
    A. <1% of causes
    B. <5% of causes
    C. <3% of causes
    D. 10% of causes
    E. 4% of causes

21. **Normal volume of testis:**
    A. 15 mL
    B. 20 mL
    C. 25 mL
    D. 30 mL
    E. 35 mL

22. **Semen analysis is considered normal according to WHO if the parameters are within which percentile:**
    A. 5th
    B. 3rd
    C. 7th
    D. 10th
    E. 15th

23. **Low ejaculate volumes indicate all except:**
    A. Retrograde ejaculation
    B. Obstruction
    C. Androgen insufficiency
    D. Advanced age
    E. Incomplete collection

24. **The effect of age on semen quality is more noted after:**
    A. 35 years
    B. 40 years
    C. 45 years
    D. 50 years
    E. 55 years

25. **The following may not correlate with severity of the ovarian hyperstimulation syndrome in assisted reproduction:**
    A. Ascites
    B. Haemoconcentration
    C. Ovarian size
    D. Acute respiratory distress syndrome (ARDS)
    E. WBC

26. **Inpatient monitoring of severe ovarian hyperstimulation includes monitoring of the following daily except:**
    A. Full blood count
    B. Haematocrit
    C. Electrolytes
    D. ABG
    E. Renal function tests

27. **Applications of anti-müllerian hormone in fertility practice include all except:**
    A. Predicting over-response to controlled ovarian hyperstimulation/OHSS
    B. Altering stimulation protocols to prevent/minimise the chance of OHSS
    C. Predicting poor response to controlled ovarian hyperstimulation
    D. Counselling couples about good response regarding multiple pregnancies
    E. Altering stimulation protocols to prevent/minimise the chance of OHSS

28. **In anovulatory infertility being treated with clomiphene how many women are considered to be clomiphene-resistant:**
    A. 15%
    B. 20%
    C. 10%
    D. 5%
    E. 3%

29. **WHO group 111—hypergonadotropic anovulation, women in this group account:**
    A. 15% causes of anovulation
    B. 10% causes
    C. 5%
    D. 3%
    E. None of the above

ANSWERS

1. **(C) 1/7**

   NICE guideline on fertility—clinical guideline 11

   Introduction: It is estimated that infertility affects 1 in 7 heterosexual couples in the UK. Since the original NICE guideline on fertility published in 2004 there has been a small increase in the prevalence of fertility problems, and a greater proportion of people now seeking help for such problems.

2. **(D) 4%**

   NICE guideline—fertility 1.3.1.1

   The results of semen analysis conducted as part of an initial assessment should be compared with the following World Health Organization reference values:
   - Semen volume: 1.5 mL or more
   - pH: 7.2 or more
   - Sperm concentration: 15 million spermatozoa per mL or more
   - Total sperm number: 39 million spermatozoa per ejaculate or more
   - Total motility (percentage of progressive motility and non-progressive motility): 40% or more motile or 32% or more with progressive motility
   - Vitality: 58% or more live spermatozoa
   - Sperm morphology (percentage of normal forms): 4% or more.

3. **(B) Woman is aged 36 years or over**

   NICE guideline definition of infertility 1.2.13.7.

   Offer an earlier referral for specialist consultation to discuss the options for attempting conception, further assessment and appropriate treatment where:
   - The woman is aged 36 years or over
   - There is a known clinical cause of infertility or a history of predisposing factors for infertility.

4. **(D) Postoperative medical management**

   Postoperative management, NICE guideline—fertility: Surgical ablation.
   - 1.7.2.1 Women with minimal or mild endometriosis who undergo laparoscopy should be offered surgical ablation or resection of endometriosis plus laparoscopic adhesiolysis because this improves the chance of pregnancy. [2004]
   - Women with ovarian endometriomas should be offered laparoscopic cystectomy because this improves the chance of pregnancy. [2004]

- Women with moderate or severe endometriosis should be offered surgical treatment because it improves the chance of pregnancy. [2004]
- Postoperative medical treatment does not improve pregnancy rates in women with moderate-to-severe endometriosis and is not recommended. [2004]

5. **(A) 2 years of unprotected sexual intercourse**

   2 years of unprotected sexual intercourse, NICE guideline—fertility. 1.8.1.3. Offer IVF treatment (see recommendations 1.11.1.3–4) to women with unexplained infertility who have not conceived after 2 years (this can include up to 1 year before their fertility investigations) of regular unprotected sexual intercourse. [new 2013]

6. **(C) Are using partner or donor sperm**

   People with unexplained infertility NICE guideline—fertility.

   Intrauterine insemination

   1.9.1.1 Consider unstimulated intrauterine insemination as a treatment option in the following groups as an alternative to vaginal sexual intercourse:
   - People who are unable to, or would find it very difficult to, have vaginal intercourse
   - Because of a clinically diagnosed physical disability or psychosexual problem who are
     - Using partner or donor sperm
   - People with conditions that require specific consideration in relation to methods of conception (for example, after sperm washing where the man is HIV positive)
   - People in same-sex relationships.

7. **(C) Past history of ovarian hyperstimulation syndrome (OHSS)**

   NICE guideline—fertility.

   1.12.3.3 When using gonadotrophins for ovarian stimulation in IVF treatment:
   - Use an individualised starting dose of follicle-stimulating hormone, based on factors that predict success, such as:
     - Age
     - BMI, presence of polycystic ovaries
   - Ovarian reserve.

8. **(A) Less than 5 mm**

   NICE guideline—fertility.

   1.12.6.2 Replacement of embryos into a uterine cavity with an endometrium of less than 5 mm thickness is unlikely to result in a pregnancy and is therefore not recommended.

9. **(C) 450 IU**

   NICE guideline—fertility.

   1.12.3.3 When using gonadotrophins for ovarian stimulation in IVF treatment do not use a dosage of follicle-stimulating hormone of more than 450 IU/day.

10. **(A) Freezing in liquid nitrogen**

    NICE guideline—fertility.

    1.16.1.9 Use freezing in liquid nitrogen vapour as the preferred cryopreservation technique for sperm.

11. **(B) 10 years**

    NICE guideline—fertility.

    16.1.12 Store cryopreserved material for an initial period of 10 years.

12. **(A) Up to 33% (one-third)**

    RCOG Green-top Guideline Number 5: Ovarian Hyperstimulation Syndrome—Incidence.

    Women should be informed that mild forms of OHSS are common, affecting up to 33% of in vitro fertilisation (IVF) cycles and that 3–8% of IVF cycles are complicated by moderate or severe OHSS.

13. **(D) Irritable bowel syndrome**

    RCOG Green-top Guideline Number 5: Ovarian Hyperstimulation Syndrome.

    Diagnosis: A diagnosis of OHSS is usually straightforward, given a history of ovarian stimulation, either by gonadotrophins or anti-oestrogens, followed by the typical symptoms of abdominal distension, abdominal pain, nausea and vomiting. Nevertheless, alternative diagnoses should always be considered, such as a complication of an ovarian cyst (torsion, haemorrhage), pelvic infection, intra-abdominal haemorrhage, ectopic pregnancy and appendicitis.

14. **(B) Severe OHSS**

    RCOG Green-top Guideline Number 5 Table 3. Classification of severity of OHSS.

    Grade Symptoms

    - Mild OHSS: Abdominal bloating, mild abdominal pain, ovarian size usually less than 8 cm*
    - Moderate OHSS: Moderate abdominal pain, nausea ± vomiting, ultrasound evidence of ascites, ovarian size usually 8–12 cm*
    - Severe OHSS: Clinical ascites (occasionally hydrothorax), oliguria, haemoconcentration, haematocrit more than 45%, hypoproteinaemia, ovarian size usually more than 12 cm*
    - Critical OHSS: Tense ascites or large hydrothorax, haematocrit more than 55%

- White cell count more than 25,000/mL
- Oliguria/anuria
- Thromboembolism, acute respiratory distress syndrome.

*ovarian size may not correlate with severity of OHSS in cases of assisted reproduction because of the effect of follicular aspiration.

15. **(A) 12 working hours of the identification of the incident and submission of an Incident Report Form within 24 working hours.**

    RCOG Green-top Guideline Number 5 on OHSS.

16. **(C) Use of GnRH antagonists**

    Women at higher risk of developing OHSS include those with polycystic ovaries, women under 30 years of age, use of GnRH agonists, development of multiple follicles during treatment, exposure to LH/hCG, and previous episodes of OHSS.

17. **(D) Hyponatraemia and hyperkalaemia**

    Hyponatraemia is seen in 56% of women with OHSS, hyperkalaemia and hyponatraemia is seen in 50% of cases.

    Prakash A, Mathur R. Ovarian hyperstimulation syndrome. The Obstetrician and Gynaecologist. 2013;15:31-5.

18. **(B) 20 mmHg**

    RCOG Green-top Guideline Number 5: OHSS 9.6.

    How should ascites or effusions should be managed? Intra-abdominal pressure may be measured via a urinary catheter with pressures greater than 20 mmHg suggestive of the need for decompression.

19. **(A) 7–10%, upper body, arterial system**

    Green-top Guideline Number 5: OHSS—thrombosis 9.7.

    The reported incidence of thrombosis with OHSS ranges between 0.7% and 10%, with an apparent preponderance of upper body sites and frequent involvement of the arterial system.

    Mechanisms contributing to thrombosis in women with OHSS include haemoconcentration, altered coagulation system and reduced venous return secondary to enlarged ovaries, ascites and immobility.

20. **(A) <1% of causes**

    Hypogonadotrophic hypogonadism is rare and accounts for less than 1% of male factor fertility problems. It results from decreased production of FSH and LH secondary to hypothalamic or pituitary dysfunction, which leads to failure of spermatogenesis and testosterone secretion by the testes. It may be congenital or acquired. Causes include craniopharyngiomas, surgery for pituitary tumours, head trauma, haemochromatosis, Kallmann syndrome and other congenital genetic syndromes of reduced gonadotrophin releasing hormone (GnRH) secretion. (Prader-Willi syndrome, Laurence-Moon-Biedl syndrome)

Karavolos S, Stewart J, Evbuomwan I, McEleny K, Aird I. Assessment of the infertile male. The Obstetrician and Gynaecologist. 2013;15:1-9.

21. **(B) 20 mL**

The scrotum should be carefully palpated with the patient standing. Testicular size and consistency should be noted. If one or other testicle is impalpable, the groin should be examined to see if it can be located. The presence and normality of the vasa differentia should be confirmed. For size measurement, an orchid meter can be used for volume estimation. A mean volume of 20 mL in the adult is considered normal.

Karavolos S , Stewart J, Evbuomwan I, McEleny K, Aird I. Assessment of the infertile male. The Obstetrician and Gynaecologist. 2013;15:1-9.

22. **(A) 5th percentile**

Semen analysis is the most important investigation of male subfertility. This is not a test for fertility but a guide for minimal standards of adequacy. What constitutes a "normal" result has been a matter of debate, and recently the WHO normal ranges for semen parameters have changed. These values represent the 5th percentile of semen characteristics of men initiating natural conception within 12 months of unprotected intercourse, in a number of different countries. It is important to remember that these are not absolute limits and should always be interpreted in conjunction with relevant clinical information to provide guidance about the prospects of a particular couple's fertility.

Refer to Karavolos S, Stewart J, Evbuomwan I, McEleny K, Aird I. Assessment of the infertile male. The Obstetrician and Gynaecologist. 2013;15:1-9.

23. **(D) Advanced age**

Fresh semen is coagulated and liquefies 15–30 minutes after ejaculation. Low ejaculate volumes of less than 1.5 mL may not buffer against vaginal acidity sufficiently. This may indicate retrograde ejaculation, obstruction, androgen deficiency, incomplete collection or an ejaculation.

Karavolos S, Stewart J, Evbuomwan I, McEleny K, Aird I. Assessment of the infertile male. The Obstetrician and Gynaecologist. 2013;15:1-9. Semen Analysis.

24. **(D) 50 years**

A UK study has shown that paternal age of more than 35 years halves the chance of achieving a pregnancy compared with a paternal age of less than 25 years. The effect of age on male fertility is more noticeable after the age of 50, with studies showing a concomitant increase in adverse outcome in the offspring. For this reason, the age of semen donors is limited to 40 years or 45 years in some countries.

Karavolos S, Stewart J, Evbuomwan I, McEleny K, Aird I. Assessment of the infertile male. The Obstetrician and Gynaecologist. 2013;15:1-9. Causes of Male Infertility.

25. **(C) Ovarian size**

    Ovarian size may not correlate to the severity of ovarian hyperstimulation due to the effect of follicular aspiration. BOX 1a.

    Prakash A, Mathur R. Ovarian hyperstimulation syndrome. The Obstetrician and Gynaecologist. 2013;15:31-5.

26. **(D) ABG**

    Table 1. Inpatient management of OHSS. ABG is done depending on the clinical features.

    Prakash A, Mathur R. Ovarian hyperstimulation syndrome. The Obstetrician and Gynaecologist. 2013;15:31-5.

27. **(D) Counselling couples about good response regarding multiple pregnancies. BOX 1**

    In conclusion (see Box 1 below), the relationship between anti-müllerian hormone (AMH) and pregnancy rates may be indirect and due to the strong and positive correlation between AMH and the number of oocytes retrieved. Current evidence does not allow AMH to be used as an independent predictor for pregnancy and further studies are needed.

    > **Box 1: Applications of anti-müllerian hormone in fertility practice**
    > - Predicting over-response to controlled ovarian hyperstimulation/OHSS
    > - Altering stimulation protocols to prevent/minimise the chance of OHSS
    > - Predicting poor response to controlled ovarian hyperstimulation
    > - Altering stimulation protocols to optimise oocyte yield in predicted poor response
    > - Counselling couples about poor response to avoid distress/disappointment

    Bhide P, Shah A, Gudi A, Homburg R. The role of anti-müllerian hormone as a predictor of ovarian function. The Obstetrician and Gynaecologist. 2012;14:161-6.

28. **(A) 15%**

    Gorthi S, Balen AH, Tang T. Current issues in ovulation induction. The Obstetrician and Gynaecologist. 2012;14:188-96.

29. **(C) 5%**

    Gorthi S, Balen AH, Tang T. Current issues in ovulation induction. The Obstetrician and Gynaecologist. 2012;14:188-96.

CHAPTER 7

Family Planning and Sexual Reproductive Health

1. **What is the incubation period for chlamydial or gonorrhoeal infection for urine sample or low vaginal swab to be accurate:**
   A. 24 hours after infection
   B. One week after infection
   C. Two weeks after infection
   D. Three weeks after infection
   E. Four weeks after infection

2. **What is the incidence of symptomatic chlamydial infection in males and females:**
   A. 50% in males and 25% in females
   B. 50% in males and 50% in females
   C. 25% in males and 50% in females
   D. 25% in males and 25% in females
   E. 25% in males and 75% in females

3. **The following are contributing factors for bacterial vaginosis infection in lower genitalia, except:**
   A. Bathing and vaginal douching
   B. Smoking
   C. Afro-Caribbean ethnicity
   D. Women fitted with intrauterine contraceptive device
   E. Sexual intercourse

4. **Which of the following drug should be avoided as first-line empirical treatment of pelvic inflammatory disease:**
   A. Doxycycline
   B. Quinolones
   C. Metronidazole
   D. Azithromycin
   E. Cefuroxime

5. **Opt-out testing for HIV offered under following circumstance:**
   A. Drug dependency
   B. Antenatal services
   C. Termination of pregnancy services
   D. Dialysis, blood donation and organ transplant services
   E. Patients accepting the test

Family Planning and Sexual Reproductive Health

6. **Characteristics features of subdermal implant, Nexplanon:**
   A. It is highly effective long-acting contraception
   B. It is radiolucent
   C. It contains 68 mg etonogestrel (ENG) dispersed in a membrane of ethylene vinyl acetate
   D. It is progestogen only implant is licensed for 3 years' use
   E. Primary mode of action is prevention of ovulation

7. **The theoretical or proven risks outweighs the advantages of using LNG-IUS contraceptive method in all the conditions except:**
   A. Positive (or unknown) anti-phospholipid antibodies
   B. Hepatocellular adenoma
   C. Migraine with aura
   D. Current or history of ischaemic heart disease
   E. History of cerebrovascular accident including TIA

8. **The risk of VTE per 10,000 healthy women over 1 year, taking combined hormonal contraception (CHC) containing ethinyl estradiol plus gestodene, desogestrel or drospirenone:**
   A. 2
   B. 5–7
   C. 6–12
   D. 9–12
   E. Less than 1

9. **The side effects may be associated with discontinuation of the contraception except:**
   A. Nausea
   B. Bloating
   C. Headache
   D. Mood swings
   E. Visual disturbance

10. **Following administration of ulipristal acetate (UPA) for emergency contraception, women continuing to use hormonal method of contraception should be advised to use additional contraceptive precautions for:**
    A. 2 days
    B. 7 days
    C. 9 days
    D. 14 days
    E. 16 days

11. **Ulipristal acetate (UPA) should not be advised as emergency contraception in women taking following drugs, except:**
    A. Liver enzyme inducing drugs
    B. Antacids
    C. Diuretics
    D. Proton pump inhibitors
    E. Histamine antagonists

12. **Indications for use of emergency contraception in women who are taking hormonal method of contraception, are all except:**
    A. If missed two or more oral combined contraceptive pill in 1 week and there has been an UPSI during that week

B. If there is an UPSI during or in the 28 days following use of liver enzyme inducing drugs
C. If desogestrel-only pill intake was delayed by more than 36 hours and there has been UPSI within 48 hours of restarting
D. If last progestogen-only injection [depot medroxyprogesterone acetate (DMPA)] was less than 14 weeks and there has been UPSI within this period
E. If hormonal method of contraception started after day 5 of the normal menstrual cycle

13. **Ulipristal acetate (UPA) as emergency contraception is recommended or used cautiously in all conditions below, except:**
    A. Uncontrolled severe asthma
    B. Hepatic dysfunction
    C. Galactose intolerance
    D. MCADD
    E. Glucose-galactose malabsorption

14. **When starting combined hormonal contraception, additional contraceptive protection should be considered when:**
    A. Women having normal menstrual cycles and the method started within day 5
    B. Women are amenorrhoea and CHC started any time
    C. CHC started on day 21 postpartum women not breastfeeding
    D. CHC started on day 5 after first or second trimester miscarriage
    E. Change over to another CHC on the day after last active COC, CTP or CVR

15. **The following conditions in women are considered as UKMEC 3/4 for use of combined hormonal contraception, except:**
    A. Migraine with aura
    B. BMI more than 35 kg/m^2
    C. Age more than 35 years
    D. Multiple risk factors for cardiovascular disease
    E. Systolic BP mare than 160 mmHg

16. **The following are the non-contraceptive health benefits with combined hormonal contraception, except:**
    A. It does not affect overall long-term mortality
    B. It reduces the risk of ovarian cancer
    C. It reduces the risk of endometrial cancer
    D. It reduces the risk of breast cancer
    E. It reduces the menopausal symptoms

17. **The following are the complications of intrauterine contraception, except:**
    A. The rate of perforation associated with IUC is around 2 in 1,000
    B. Risk expulsion is around 1 in 20 in the first year of use
    C. After removal of IUC, fertility is delayed

D. The ovarian cysts may occur when using LNG-IUS
E. The risk of developing pelvic inflammatory disease after IUC insertion is less than 1 in 100

18. If a woman becomes pregnant while using IUC and an intrauterine pregnancy is confirmed, when is the best time to remove the IUC:
    A. Before 6 weeks of gestation
    B. Before 8 weeks of gestation
    C. Before 10 weeks of gestation
    D. Before 12 weeks of gestation
    E. Before 14 weeks of gestation

19. What is the primary mode of action of progestogen-only pill (POP) that contributes to its contraceptive effect:
    A. Inhibits of ovulation
    B. Increases volume and viscosity of cervical mucus
    C. Hinders implantation by causing endometrial changes
    D. Reduces in cilia activity in fallopian tube
    E. Causes inflammatory changes in the endometrial cavity

20. Women with unscheduled bleeding during the use of a progestogen-only injectable contraceptive, treated with:
    A. Combined oral contraceptive for 3 months
    B. Progestogen-only pill for 3 months
    C. Mefenamic acid 500 mg tds for 3 months
    D. The scheduled injectable given earlier than its due period
    E. No treatment is needed

21. Long-acting reversible contraception of choice in women with sickle cell disease is:
    A. Progestogen-only pill
    B. Progestogen-only implant
    C. Progestogen-only injectable
    D. Intrauterine contraception
    E. Combined hormonal contraception

22. Which is the most appropriate site for the insertion of subdermal implant:
    A. Mid part of upper arm
    B. Just above the medial epicondyle of humerus in non-dominant arm
    C. 8–10 cm above lateral epicondyle of humerus in non-dominant arm
    D. 8–10 cm above medial epicondyle of humerus in non-dominant arm
    E. 10 cm below the medial epicondyle of humerus

23. Which one of the following occlusion techniques of vasectomy has lower likelihood of recanalisation:
    A. Cauterisation and division of vas deferens
    B. Fascial interposition after cauterisation
    C. Ligation of divided vas deferens
    D. Insertion of intra vas devices or plugs
    E. Fulguration of lumen after division of vas deferens

24. **When is the optimal timing for post-vasectomy semen analysis (PVSA) to detect early failure:**
    A. 6 weeks after the procedure
    B. 8 weeks
    C. 10 weeks
    D. 12 weeks
    E. 14 weeks

25. **After laparoscopic tubal occlusion, women using combined hormonal contraception should ideally:**
    A. Stop using the contraception before the procedure
    B. Stop using contraception immediately after the procedure
    C. Continue for 7 days after the procedure
    D. Continue for 28 days after the procedure
    E. Use additional contraceptive protection

26. **The failure rate of laparoscopic tubal occlusion with Filshie clips, in 10 years:**
    A. Less than 1 per 1,000 procedures
    B. 2–3 per 1,000 procedures
    C. 5–8 per 1,000 procedures
    D. 10–20 per 1,000 procedures
    E. More than 20 per 1,000 procedures

27. **A confirmatory imaging test after insertion of intra-fallopian micro-inserts should be undertaken:**
    A. Within 1 month by X-ray pelvis
    B. Within 2 months with X-ray pelvis or transvaginal ultrasound
    C. Within 3 months by hysterosalpingogram (HSG)
    D. After 3 months by X-ray pelvis or transvaginal ultrasound
    E. After 4 months by transvaginal ultrasound

28. **If female condoms are used consistently and correctly, they are:**
    A. 80% effective
    B. 85% effective
    C. 90% effective
    D. 95% effective
    E. 98% effective.

29. **To diagnose menopause in perimenopausal women using hormonal contraception, one of the following statement is correct:**
    A. Amenorrhoea is a reliable indicator of ovarian failure
    B. Serum follicle stimulating hormone (FSH) more than 30 IU/L indicates menopause in women using progestogen-only method
    C. Two readings of serum FSH more than 30 IU/L indicates menopause in women using progestogen-only methods
    D. In women under 50 years using combined hormonal contraception, raised serum FSH indicates ovarian failure
    E. Raised serum FSH is a reliable indicator of ovarian failure.

30. **Women who have their LNG-IUS inserted for contraception at the age of 45 years or over, can use the device for:**
    A. 4 years
    B. 5 years
    C. 7 years
    D. Remove at the of age 50 years
    E. Not advisable to use after 45 years of age

31. **A 22-year-old has UPSI (unprotected sexual intercourse) in her night out. She recently was diagnosed with pelvic inflammatory disease (PID) and had taken ulipristal acetate (UPA) a week back for similar episode. She is requesting for a morning after pill. What would you offer?**
    A. Levonorgestrel
    B. Ulipristal acetate
    C. Copper T
    D. All are suitable
    E. None

32. **A 28-year-old comes to you requesting for emergency contraception, she had UPSI 4 days back. She fears examination and requesting not to be examined if possible. What would be most suitable advice for her?**
    A. Levonorgestrel 3 mg
    B. UPA 30 mg
    C. Copper T
    D. Double dose of COCP
    E. Levonorgestrel 1.5 mg

33. **Levonorgestrel, which is the incorrect statement:**
    A. Acts by preventing follicular rupture or cause luteal dysfunction
    B. Inhibits ovulation
    C. Is most effective if given closer to ovulation
    D. Used as emergency contraception (EC)
    E. Is a progestogen hormone

34. **Which is the incorrect statement regarding UPA**
    A. A progesterone receptor modulator
    B. Recommended dose as EC is 20 mg single oral dose
    C. Mechanism of action is inhibition or delay of ovulation
    D. Can prevent ovulation even after the LH surge has started
    E. None

35. **Correct statement regarding EVRA transdermal patches:**
    A. Contains norelgestromin and ethinyl estradiol
    B. EVRA can be used as an HRT
    C. There is no patch-free week
    D. Should be started within 1 week of childbirth for complete protection if the women do not intend to breastfeed
    E. None

36. **Incorrect statement regarding CHC:**
    A. There is a small increase in the risk of cervical cancer which is related to duration of use
    B. CHC does not appear to have a negative effect on overall mortality
    C. CHC is associated with a reduction in ovarian cancer
    D. CHC is associated with a reduction in endometrial cancer
    E. None

37. **Incorrect statement regarding progestogen-only pills (POP):**
    A. Cerazette contains desogestrel and has a window period of 12 hours in-comparison to other POPs, which has window period of 3 hours
    B. Primary mode of action of Cerazette is inhibition of ovulation
    C. All POP's if correctly used are more than 99% effective
    D. It is recommended that women weighing more than 70 kg should take two traditional POPs a day
    E. None

38. **POP is UKMEC 4 category for:**
    A. Current VTE
    B. Hereditary thrombophilia
    C. Current IHD
    D. Current breast cancer
    E. Malignant liver tumour

39. **IUD as a contraceptive is used by _____ % of the UK population.**
    A. 1%
    B. 5%
    C. 10%
    D. 15%
    E. 25%

40. **The risk of uterine perforation during insertion of IUD is:**
    A. 2 per 1,000
    B. 5 per 1,000
    C. 1 per 100
    D. 5 per 100
    E. 10 per 1,000

41. **Correct statement IUD**
    A. Prior to insertion, all women having a Mirena/Cu-IUD should be screened for sexually transmitted infections
    B. LNG-IUS fitted over the age of 45 years can be left in situ for 7 years
    C. LNG-IUS is not suitable for women with epilepsy on liver enzyme-inducing drugs
    D. LNG-IUS use in women with breast cancer is UKMEC Category 3
    E. Cu-IUD primarily works by preventing implantation

42. **Incorrect statement regarding progestogen-only implant:**
    A. Implant contains 68 mg etonogestrel
    B. Licensed for 3 years
    C. Release rate decreases with time
    D. Not affected by concomitant use of enzyme-inducing drugs
    E. There is no restriction on its use in women with BMI more than 30 kg/m^2

43. **Incorrect statement regarding progestogen-only injectable contraception:**
    A. Used by 3% of the women aged 16–49 years in UK
    B. Primary mode of action is inhibition of ovulation
    C. Cumulative pregnancy rate is less than 4 in 1,000
    D. There can be delay in return of fertility following discontinuation
    E. Up to 90% are amenorrhoeic after 6 months of use

44. **Depot medroxyprogesterone acetate (DMPA):**
    A. Licensed for 12 weeks
    B. There is an association between DMPA use and weight gain
    C. Most common reason for discontinuation is changes in bleeding pattern
    D. DMPA is associated with a small loss in BMD
    E. Efficacy of DMPA is affected by the use of non-liver enzyme inducing antibiotics hence use of additional non-hormonal contraception is advised

45. **Choose the incorrect statement regarding Sayana Press Retard:**
    A. Is combined hormonal form of injectable contraception licensed for subcutaneous use
    B. Primary mode of action is preventing ovulation
    C. It has the advantage over IM DMPA in patients with bleeding disorders
    D. The return of fertility is similar to IM DMPA
    E. None

46. **Incorrect statement regarding male sterilization is:**
    A. Failure rate of male sterilization is 1 in 2,000
    B. Minimal invasive approach should be used
    C. Cauterization followed by division of the vas deferens is the recommended method
    D. Special clearance can be given when less than 10,000 non-motile sperm/mL are observed in a fresh semen sample post-vasectomy
    E. At the age of 40–49 years 30% of males are sterilized

47. **Incorrect statement regarding female sterilization:**
    A. Does not need anaesthesia
    B. Is a permanent procedure
    C. Additional contraception is required until tubal occlusion is confirmed by imaging at least 3 months after the procedure
    D. Failure rate is approximately 1 in 500 at 5 years
    E. None

48. **In UK Essure recommends Hysterosalpingogram (HSG) should be used as first-line of imaging in following circumstance except:**
    A. There was concern regarding possible perforation
    B. There was difficulty identifying the tubal ostia

C. There was uncertainty by the professional regarding placement of the micro-insert
D. Procedure time more than 15 minutes
E. None

49. **UKMEC category for a woman with positive antiphospholipid antibodies intending to have a Nexplanon inserted:**
    A. UKMEC 1
    B. UKMEC 2
    C. UKMEC 3
    D. UKMEC 4
    E. Undefined

50. **Risk of transmission of HIV from HIV positive male to female is negligible when all the following criteria are met except:**
    A. Man is compliant with HAART
    B. The plasma viral load is less than 50 copies/mL for more than 3 months
    C. There are no other infections present
    D. Unprotected intercourse is limited to the time of ovulation
    E. None.

ANSWERS

1. **(C) Two weeks after infection**
   The incubation period for chlamydia and gonorrhoea is up to 2 weeks. If patients are tested within the incubation periods of these infections their test results could be falsely negative. (*e-SRH 11—testing for sexually transmitted and genital infections. FSRH.org*).

2. **(A) 50% in males and 25% in females**
   (*e-SRH 11—testing for sexually transmitted and genital infections. FSRH.org*).

3. **(E) Sexual intercourse**
   Bacterial vaginosis (BV) is sexually related rather that transmitted, the symptoms often get worse immediately following sexual intercourse and following menstruation, all other factors contribute for vaginal commensal to proliferate such as *Gardnerella vaginalis*, *Mobiluncus* species and anaerobes like *Prevotella*. (*e-SRH 12—Abnormal vulvovaginal symptoms. FSRH.org*).

4. **(B) Quinolones**
   Quinolones should be avoided in patients who are at high risk of gonococcal pelvic inflammatory disease (PID) because of increasing quinolone resistance in the UK. Quinolones should also be avoided as first-line empirical treatment for PID in areas where more than 5% of PID is caused by quinolone resistant *Neisseria gonorrhoeae*. (*Management of PID: Green-top Guidelines Number 32*).

5. **(B) Antenatal services**
   British Association for Sexual Health and HIV (BASHH) and British HIV Association (BHIVA) recommend that HIV testing should be offered routinely in the following circumstances on opt-out basis to increase the likelihood of patients agreeing to test: GUM and sexual health clinic, antenatal services, termination of pregnancy services, dialysis, blood donation and organ transplant services and healthcare services for those diagnosed with tuberculosis, Hepatitis B, Hepatitis C and lymphoma. (*e-SRH 13; HIV testing FSRH.org*).

6. **(B) It is radiolucent**
   Implanon is replaced by Nexplanon. The only difference between the two is Nexplanon is radio-opaque. (*Progesterone-only Implants: FSRH.org*).

7. **(C) Migraine with aura**
   Migraine with aura is UKMEC 2 for all progesterone-only contraception, i.e. benefits with these contraception outweighs the risks. (*UK Medical Eligibility Criteria 9 UKMEC for contraception use, FSRH.org*).

8. **(D) 9–12**

    FSRH statement on VTE and hormonal contraception

	Risk of venous thromboembolism (VTE) per 10,000 healthy women over 1 year
Non-contraceptive users and not pregnant	2
Combined hormonal contraception (CHC) containing ethinyl estradiol plus levonorgestrel, norgestimate or norethisterone	5–7
CHC containing etonogestrel (ring) or norelgestromin (patch)	6–12
CHC containing ethinyl estradiol plus gestodene, desogestrel or drospirenone	9–12

9. **(E) Visual disturbance**

    All are side effects of combined methods. Compared to pill users, CTP users experience more breast discomfort, dysmenorrhoea, nausea and vomiting. CVR users report less nausea, acne, irritability and depression than pill users, but experience more vaginal irritation and discharge (*Combined hormonal contraception, e-modules, FSRH.org*).

10. **(D) 14 days**

    Following administration of UPA, women continuing to use a hormonal method of contraception should be advised to use additional contraceptive precautions for 14 days [9 days for progestogen-only pill (POP), 16 days for Qlaira]. (*Emergency contraception, FSRH.org*).

11. **(C) Diuretics**

    Women taking liver enzyme-inducing drugs should be advised not to use UPA during or within 28 days of stopping this medication. Women should be advised not to use UPA if they are currently taking drugs which increase gastric pH, e.g. antacids, histamine H_2 antagonists and proton pump inhibitors. (*Emergency contraception, FSRH.org*).

12. **(D) If last progestogen-only injection [depot medroxyprogesterone acetate (DMPA)] was less than 14 weeks and there has been UPSI within this period**

    (Refer to Emergency contraception, FSRH.org).

13. **(D) Medium chain acyl-CoA dehydrogenase deficiency (MCADD)**

    Use of UPA is not recommended in severe asthma insufficiently controlled by oral glucocorticoids. In women with hepatic dysfunction, hereditary problems such as galactose intolerance, lactate deficiency or glucose-galactose malabsorption, UPA used with caution. After intake of UPA, breastfeeding is not recommended for up to 36 hours. (*Emergency contraception, FSRH.org*).

14. **(B) Women are amenorrhoea and CHC started any time**

    Additional contraceptive protection is required if CHC is started after day 5 of the cycle, after day 21 postpartum, women who are amenorrhoeic and after day 5 post-abortion. (*Combined hormonal contraception guidance, FSRH.org*).

15. **(C) Age more than 35 years**

    Age alone is not a risk factor to use combined hormonal contraception. CHC can used up to the age of 50 if there are no other risk factors. Use of CHC in women aged more than 35 years who smoke is not recommended. (*Combined hormonal contraception guidance, FSRH.org*).

16. **(D) It reduces the risk of breast cancer**

    Women can be advised that CHC unlikely to affect overall long-term mortality nor have negative effect on overall mortality. The risk of developing or dying from ovarian and endometrial cancer is reduced with use of COC. COC use also decreases the risk of colorectal cancer. CHC maintain the bone health. COC can be used to treat dysmenorrhoea and HMB. A large meta-analysis of case-control studies showed an increased risk of breast cancer whilst using COC which is approximately an increase of 24% above the background risk. (*Combined hormonal contraception guidance, FSRH.org*).

17. **(C) After removal of IUC, fertility is delayed**

    The risk of expulsion with IUC is around 1 in 20 and is most common in the first year of use, particularly within 3 months of insertion. There is no need to delay insertion of an IUC post-abortion providing a woman has been informed of the small increased risk of expulsion. Although ovarian cysts may occur when using the LNG-IUS, most cysts are asymptomatic and resolve spontaneously. The rate of uterine perforation associated with IUC is up to 2 per 1,000 insertions and is approximately six-fold higher in breastfeeding women. Return of fertility after IUC use is generally similar to fertility rates after discontinuation of oral contraceptives and barrier methods. Cu-IUD users with recurrent bacterial vaginosis or vulvovaginal candida may wish to consider an alternative method of contraception. (*IUC guidance, FSRH.org*).

18. **(D) Before 12 weeks of gestation**

    If a woman becomes pregnant while using IUC, the site of the pregnancy should be determined by ultrasound scan and advice given regarding the removal of intrauterine method before 12 weeks. If LNG IUS is used, ectopic pregnancy should be ruled out and remove the IUS and offer termination of pregnancy. (*IUC guidance, FSRH.org*).

19. **(B) Increases volume and viscosity of cervical mucus**

   The POPs have several independent modes of action that contribute to its contraceptive effect. The main action is increase in volume and viscosity of cervical mucus preventing sperm penetration into the upper reproductive tract. The other modes of action include suppression of ovulation, endometrial changes that hinder implantation and reduction of cilia activity in the fallopian tube that slows the passage of an ovum. (*Progestogen-only Pill Guidance, FSRH.org*).

20. **(A) Combined oral contraceptive for 3 months**

   Women who are medically eligible can be offered a COC for 3 months or mefenamic acid 500 mg TDS for 5 days to treat unscheduled bleeding with progestogen-only injectable. (*Progestogen-only Injectable Guidance, FSRH.org*).

21. **(C) Progestogen-only injectable**

   Depot medroxyprogesterone acetate (DMPA) is a contraceptive option for women with sickle cell disease and may reduce the severity of sickle crisis pain. For women taking antiepileptic or antiretroviral drugs that induce liver enzymes DMPA may be an appropriate method of contraception because its efficacy is unaffected. (*Progestogen-only Injectable Guidance, FSRH.org*).

22. **(D) 8–10 cm above medial epicondyle of humerus in non-dominant arm**

   The SPC advises that the implant should be inserted 8–10 cm up the arm from the medial epicondyle. Because of natural variation in arm lengths the guideline development group agreed that 8–10 cm is not always the ideal distance, and that as a general guide the insertion site should be one-third of the way up the arm from the elbow. Care should be taken to avoid deep insertion into muscle, nerves or blood vessels. (*Progestogen-only Implant, FSRH.org*).

23. **(A) Cauterisation and division of vas deferens**

   There is consensus in the literature that cauterisation is an effective vasectomy method. Two cohort studies that examined cauterisation as a vasectomy technique reported a failure rate of 0.8% and 0.38%, respectively, and an 85% probability of achieving azoospermia at 12 weeks. (*Male and female sterilisation, FSRH.org*).

24. **(D) 12 weeks**

   Evidence suggests that 12 weeks post-vasectomy is the optimal timing to schedule the first PVSA. Earlier or later testing is acceptable taking into account that earlier testing increases the probability of additional tests and later testing prolongs the need for additional contraception. (*Male and female sterilisation, FSRH.org*).

25. **(C) Continue for 7 days after the procedure**

    Theoretically, CHC could be stopped at the time of laparoscopic tubal occlusion if it has been consistently and correctly used in the previous 7 days. However, the multidisciplinary guideline development group considered it a safe and simple approach to advise that CHC (i.e. COC, vaginal ring, transdermal patch) should be continued for at least 7 days. If sterilisation is scheduled for the hormone-free interval or day 1 of a cycle of CHC following the hormone-free interval, CHC should be restarted. Alternatively, the hormone-free interval can be omitted and CHC continued for a minimum of 7 days after sterilisation. (*Male and female sterilisation, FSRH.org*).

26. **(B) 2–3 per 1,000 procedures**

    Late failures resulting in a pregnancy can occur any time after tubal occlusion. The lifetime risk of laparoscopic tubal occlusion failure, using a mix of occlusion methods, is estimated to be 1 in 200. The longest period of available follow-up data for the most commonly used method in the UK, the Filshie clip, suggests a failure rate of 2–3 per 1,000 procedures at 10 years. (*Male and female sterilisation, FSRH.org*).

27. **(D) After 3 months by X-ray pelvis or transvaginal ultrasound**

    The micro-inserts elicit a benign tissue response (fibrosis) resulting in the permanent occlusion of each tube after approximately 3 months. A confirmatory imaging test should be undertaken 3 months after the insertion of intra-fallopian micro-inserts. This may be via X-ray or transvaginal ultrasound scanning (TVUSS) in the first instance, followed by hysterosalpingogram (HSG) in selected patients where X-ray/TVUSS cannot confirm satisfactory placement. Additional contraception is required until successful placement of the micro-inserts and tubal occlusion is confirmed. (*Male and female sterilisation, FSRH.org*).

28. **(D) 95% effective**

    Male condoms are 98% effective and female condoms are 95% effective at preventing pregnancy but only when used consistently and correctly. (*Barrier contraception, FSRH.org*).

29. **(B) Serum follicle stimulating hormone (FSH) more than 30 IU/L indicates menopause in women using progestogen-only method**

    Women using exogenous hormones should be advised that amenorrhoea is not a reliable indicator of ovarian failure. In women using contraceptive hormones, FSH levels may be used to help diagnose the menopause, but should be restricted to women over the age of 50 years and to those using progestogen-only methods. FSH is not a reliable indicator of ovarian failure in women using combined hormones, even if measured during the hormone-free interval. Women over the age of 50 years who are amenorrhoeic and wish to stop POC can have their FSH levels checked. If the level is more than or equal to 30 IU/L the FSH should be repeated after 6 weeks. If the second FSH level is more than or equal to 30 IU/L contraception can be stopped after 1 year. (*Contraception for women over 40 years, FSRH.org*).

30. **(C) 7 years**

    Women who have had an LNG-IUS inserted at the age of 45 years or over may continue to use the method for 7 years if their bleeding pattern is acceptable. NICE guidance advises that if women have an LNG-IUS inserted at or after the age of 45 years and are amenorrhoeic they may continue to use the LNG-IUS until they are postmenopausal. (*Contraception for women over 40 years, FSRH.org*).

31. **(A) Levonorgestrel**

    As she recently had (UPA) she is not suitable for it, guidelines recommends avoiding it twice in a cycle. There is no information about treatment for PID hence Copper T should be avoided.

32. **(B) UPA 30 mg**

    Refer to FSRH guidance August, 2011: Emergency Contraception.

33. **(C) Is most effective if given closer to ovulation**

    Refer to FSRH guidance August, 2011: Emergency Contraception.

34. **(B) Recommended dose as EC is 20 mg single oral dose is incorrect statement.**

    Refer to FSRH Guidance August, 2011: Emergency Contraception. Recommended dose of UPA as EC is 30 mg single oral dose.

35. **(A) Contains norelgestromin and ethinyl estradiol**

    Refer to SPC product information. May 2015. EVRA is a 20 cm² transdermal patch contains 6 mg norelgestromin and 600 µg ethinyl estradiol (EE). Each patch is used for 1 week from day 1 (first day of the menses), should be changed on day 8 and day 15. Fourth week is patch-free week.

36. **(A) There is a small increase in the risk of cervical cancer which is related to duration of use**

    Refer to FSRH guidelines on combined hormonal contraceptive October, 2011 (updated August, 2012).

37. **(D) It is recommended that women weighing more than 70 kg should take two traditional POPs a day**

    Refer to Faculty of Sexual and Reproductive healthcare clinical guidance. Progestogen-only Pills June, 2009.

38. **(D) Current breast cancer**

    Refer to UKMEC, 2015. The only UKMEC 4 category for POPs is current breast cancer. Current VTE is UKMEC 2 and hereditary thrombophilia

Family Planning and Sexual Reproductive Health

is UKMEC 2. Current IHD is UKMEC 2 for initiation and UKMEC 3 for continuation. Malignant liver tumour is UKMEC 3.

39. **(B) 5%**

Refer to FSRH Clinical Guidance: Intrauterine Contraception (November, 2007).

Failure rate are very low 1-2%. Primary mode of action of a Cu-IUD is prevention of fertilisation. The risk of expulsion is 1 in 20 and is most common in the first year of use, particularly within 3 months of insertion.

40. **(A) 2 per 1,000**

Refer to FSRH Clinical Guidance: Intrauterine Contraception. (November, 2007).

Failure rate are very low 1-2%. Primary mode of action of a Cu-IUD is prevention of fertilisation. The risk of expulsion is 1 in 20 and is most common in the first year of use, particularly within 3 months of insertion.

41. **(B) LNG-IUS fitted over the age of 45 years can be left in situ for 7 years**

Refer to FSRH Clinical Guidance: Intrauterine Contraception. (November, 2007).

Only women who are symptomatic or are at risk should be screened for STI. LNG-IUS use in woman with breast cancer is UKMEC Category 4 and Cu-IUD primarily works by preventing fertilization.

42. **(D) Not affected by concomitant use of enzyme-inducing drugs**

Refer to FSRH Guidance (February, 2014). Progestogen-only Implants.

43. **(C) Cumulative pregnancy rate is less than 4 in 1,000**

Refer to FSRH Guidance (February, 2014) Progestogen-only Implants.

Up to 70% of DMPA users are amenorrhoeic at 1 year of use.

Up to 50% discontinue by 1 year of use and the most common reason for discontinuation is changes to bleeding pattern.

44. **(E) Efficacy of DMPA is affected by the use of non-liver enzyme inducing antibiotics hence use of additional non-hormonal contraception is advised**

Refer to FSRH Guidance (February, 2014) Progestogen-only Injectable Contraception (December, 2014, updated March, 2015).

45. **(A) Is combined hormonal form of injectable contraception licensed for subcutaneous use**

Refer to FSRH subcutaneous depot medroxyprogesterone acetate; June, 2013.

Sayana Press Retard is a progestogen-only injectable contraceptive licensed for subcutaneous use. Contains 104 mg of medroxyprogesterone acetate and administered every 13 weeks ± 7 days.

46. **(D) Special clearance can be given when less than 10,000 non-motile sperm/mL are observed in a fresh semen sample post-vasectomy**

    Refer to FSRH Guidance (September. 2014): Male and female sterilisation. The RCOG guidance published in 2004 suggested a threshold of 10,000 non-motile sperm/mL whereas the updated document suggests a threshold of 100,000 non-motile sperm/mL.

47. **(B) Is a permanent procedure**

    Refer to FSRH Guidance (September, 2014): Male and Female sterilisation.

48. **(E) None**

    Refer to FSRH Guidance (September, 2014): Male and female sterilisation.

    Also it should be the first-line of imaging if:
    - The micro-insert placement with 0 or more than 8 trailing coils
    - Unusual post-procedural pain
    - If X-ray or TVUSS is equivocal or unsatisfactory.

49. **(C) UKMEC 3**

    Refer to UKMEC 2015.

50. **(B) The plasma viral load is less than 50 copies/mL for more than 3 months**

    Refer to BHIVA guidelines on management of HIV infection in pregnant women 2012. Plasma viral load should be less than 50 copies for more than 6 months.

CHAPTER 8

Early Pregnancy Care

1. **What percentage of partial moles are triploid in origin?**
   A. 10%
   B. 20%
   C. 50%
   D. 75%
   E. 90%

2. **What percentage of complete moles arise from dispermic fertilization?**
   A. 10–20%
   B. 20–25%
   C. 75–80%
   D. 90%
   E. 100%

3. **Risk of woman with partial molar pregnancy needing chemotherapy is:**
   A. 0.5%
   B. 1–2%
   C. 5%
   D. 10%
   E. 15%

4. **Need for chemotherapy following complete mole is:**
   A. 0.5%
   B. 1%
   C. 5%
   D. 15%
   E. 25%

5. **Cure rate for women with FIGO 2000 score less than 6 is nearly:**
   A. 25%
   B. 50%
   C. 75%
   D. 100%
   E. None

6. **History indicated cervical cerclage is performed:**
   A. 12–14 weeks
   B. In asymptomatic women
   C. Cervical length less than 25 mm
   D. A + B
   E. A + C

7. **Ultrasound indicated cervical cerclage is performed:**
   A. 10–12 weeks
   B. 12–14 weeks
   C. 18–20 weeks
   D. 12–20 weeks
   E. 14–24 weeks

8. **Contraindications to cervical cerclage are all except:**
   A. Active labour
   B. Clinical evidence of chorioamnionitis
   C. PPROM
   D. Vaginal bleeding
   E. None

9. **Ultrasound indicated cerclage is offered:**
   A. Primigravid with short cervix
   B. Woman with history of preterm labour
   C. Incidental finding of cervix of less than 25 mm
   D. Cervical funneling
   E Women with history of preterm labour and cervical length less than 25 mm

10. **Risk of recurrence of molar pregnancy in a woman with previous molar is:**

A. 1 in 10	B. 1 in 25
C. 1 in 55	D. 1 in 100
E. 1 in 250	

11. **Risk of relapse following successful treatment of trophoblastic disease in a low risk disease is:**

A. 0.1%	B. 1%
C. 2%	D. 5%
E. 10%	

12. **Rate of molar pregnancy is approximately:**

A. 1 in 100 live births	B. 1 in 500 live births
C. 1 in 700 live births	D. 1 in 7,000 live births
E. 1 in 10,000 live births	

13. **In what percentage women no identifiable risk factor for ectopic is found?**

A. 1%	B. 10%
C. 25%	D. 50%
E. 75%	

14. **Bagel sign is seen:**
    A. Hydatidiform mole
    B. Chocolate cyst
    C. Appendicitis
    D. Retained products of conception
    E. Ectopic pregnancy

15. **Negative sliding sign is an ultrasound feature of:**

A. Tubal ectopic	B. Cervical ectopic
C. Interstitial ectopic	D. Abdominal ectopic
E. Caesarean section scar ectopic	

16. **Interstitial line sign is seen in:**
    A. Tubal pregnancy
    B. Cervical pregnancy
    C. Caesarean scar pregnancy
    D. Heterotopic pregnancy
    E. Interstitial pregnancy.

17. **Women who had rubella vaccine is advised**
    A. To try pregnancy whenever she wishes
    B. To avoid pregnancy for 1 month
    C. To avoid pregnancy for 3 months
    D. To avoid pregnancy for 6 months
    E. None

18. **Incorrect statement regarding complications of abortion is:**
    A. Risk of uterine rupture associated with medical abortion at late gestation is less than 1 in 1,000
    B. Risk of bleeding requiring blood transfusion in early abortion is less than 1 in 1,000
    C. Risk of bleeding requiring blood transfusion in late abortion is 4 in 1,000
    D. Cervical trauma associated with surgical abortion is 1 in 100
    E. Risk of failure to end the pregnancy and there by necessitating another procedure is less than 1 in 1,000

ANSWERS

1. **(E) 90%**
   Refer to GTG Number 38.
2. **(B) 20–25%**
   Refer to GTG Number 38.
   Complete moles usually 75–80% arise as a consequence of duplication of a single sperm following fertilization of an empty ovum. Some complete moles 20–25% can arise after dispermic fertilization of an empty ovum.
3. **(A) 0.5%**
   Refer to GTG Number 38.
4. **(D) 15%**
   Refer to GTG Number 38.
5. **(D) 100%**
   Refer to GTG Number 38.
   In the UK, there is an effective registration and treatment programme. The programme has achieved impressive results, with cure rate of 98–100% and low (5–8%) chemotherapy rates. The cure rate for women with score less than 6 is almost 100%, while women with scores 7 or more is 95%.
6. **(D) A + B**
   Refer to GTG Number 60.
7. **(E) 14–24 weeks**
   Refer to GTG Number 60.
8. **(E) None**
   Refer to GTG Number 60.
9. **(E) Women with history of preterm labour and cervical length less than 25 mm**
   Refer to GTG Number 60.
10. **(C) 1 in 55**
    Refer to TOG 2008 volume 10 issue 1.
    Risk of recurrence is 1 in 55 with one previous molar pregnancy and 1 in 10 in 2 previous molar pregnancies.
11. **(C) 2%**
    Refer to TOG 2008 volume 10 issue 1.
    The risk of relapse is 2% for a low-risk woman and 3% for a high-risk women treated with EMA/CO chemotherapy. Recurrence usually happens within first 12 months.
12. **(C) 1 in 700 live births**
    Refer to TOG 2008 volume 10 issue 1.

13. **(D) 50%**
    Refer to TOG 2015 volume 17 issue 3.
    Recognised risk factors for ectopic are smoking, pelvic inflammatory disease, previous ectopic pregnancy, ART and previous tubal surgery. In the UK, 11 maternal deaths were attributed to ectopic pregnancy in the last triennial Centre for Maternal and Child Enquiries (CMACE) report.

14. **(E) Ectopic pregnancy**
    Refer to TOG 2015 volume 17 issue 3.
    Transvaginal approach is now the gold standard for diagnosing ectopic pregnancy. Using this approach over 70% of ectopic pregnancies may be diagnosed at the time of the presentation and over 90% may be visualized after a follow-up scan. The ultrasound features include:
    An adnexal mass with hyperechoic ring around the gestational sac (Bagel sign).
    A homogenous mass seen separate to the ovary (Blob sign).

15. **(B) Cervical ectopic**
    Refer to TOG 2015 volume 17 issue 3.
    Ultrasound criteria currently used to make a diagnosis of cervical pregnancy are:
    An empty uterus
    A barrel-shaped cervix
    A gestational sac or trophoblastic mass below the level of the internal os
    A negative "sliding sign"
    Evidence of sustained peri-trophoblastic circulation on colour Doppler examination.

16. **(E) Interstitial pregnancy**
    Refer to TOG 2015 volume 17 issue 3.
    Interstitial pregnancy is when implantation occurs in the interstitial portion of the fallopian tube, occurs in 1–6% of ectopic pregnancies. The "interstitial line sign" seen in interstitial ectopic pregnancy involves visualising the thin echogenic line of the endometrial cavity and following this along to the periphery of the interstitial sac. This sign has 80% sensitivity and 98% specificity. Interstitial ectopic pregnancy presents late in pregnancy.

17. **(B) To avoid pregnancy for 1 month**
    Refer to NICE clinical guidelines on fertility.

18. **(E) Risk of failure to end the pregnancy and there by necessitating another procedure is less than 1 in 1,000**
    Refer to RCOG: Care of women requesting-induced abortion (November, 2011).
    The risk of needing repeat procedure due to failure to end the pregnancy is less than 1 in 100.

CHAPTER 9

Gynaeoncology

1. **Which one of the following is true about human papillomavirus (HPV) vaccine**
   A. HPV vaccine is 100% efficacious in preventing the cervical cancer
   B. Gardasil vaccine is given as a three dose schedule
   C. Immunocompromised girls can be given same number of doses as recommended for immunocompetent
   D. Cervarix (bivalent) vaccine is more efficacious than Gardasil (quadrivalent) vaccine
   E. HPV vaccine is an inactivated vaccine but not recommended in pregnancy

2. **The following are contributing factors that cause the HPV infection that can lead to development of cervical cancer, except**
   A. Persistent high risk HPV infection
   B. Alcohol
   C. Smoking
   D. Increasing number of full term pregnancies
   E. HIV infection

3. **There is an increased rate of obstetric complications after the treatment of cervical intraepithelial neoplasia (CIN) except:**
   A. Low birth weight
   B. Preterm delivery
   C. Perinatal mortality
   D. Increased rate of caesarean section
   E. Mid trimester miscarriage

4. **Women who had treatment for CIN, have increased risk of preterm delivery in future pregnancy except:**
   A. If treated for high grade lesion
   B. If women had two excision treatments
   C. If the excision loop was more than 10 mm
   D. If women had knife conisation
   E. If women had ablative technique

5. **Five year survival rate for advanced ovarian cancer is:**
   A. 10–20% B. 20–30%
   C. 30–40% D. 40–50%
   E. 50–60%

6. **Hereditary gynaecological cancers manifest in following conditions except:**
   A. Li-Fraumeni syndrome B. Cowden syndrome
   C. Peutz-Jeghers syndrome D. Lynch syndrome
   E. Triple X syndrome

7. **Ideal age to offer risk reducing bilateral salpingo-oophorectomy in women with *BRCA1* and *2* mutation carriers is:**
   A. Perimenopausal age B. Less than 50 years
   C. Less than 45 years D. Less than 40 years
   E. Less than 35 years

8. **The risk of primary peritoneal cancer in women with *BRCA1* and *2* mutation carriers after undergoing risk reducing bilateral salpingo-oophorectomy is:**
   A. Less than 1% B. 1–5%
   C. 5–10% D. 10–15%
   E. More than 20%

9. **The following fertility sparing treatments could be considered in gynaecological cancers except:**
   A. Radical vaginal trachelectomy in early adenocarcinoma of endocervix
   B. Neoadjuvant chemotherapy and loop excision in stage I cervical cancer
   C. Conservative surgery in stage IA germ cell tumours
   D. High dose of progestogens in treatment of stage IA endometrioid endometrial cancer
   E. Ovarian transposition in women with cervical cancer undergoing pelvic irradiation

10. **The following treatment options can be considered in the morbidly obese women with endometrial cancer to reduce the postoperative morbidities:**
    A. Minimal access surgery preferred to open laparotomy
    B. Hysterectomy along with apronectomy in open procedures to prevent wound infection
    C. Primary radiotherapy
    D. Chemotherapy
    E. High dose progestogens

11. **The characteristic features of borderline ovarian tumours are, except:**
    A. Seen in younger age group
    B. Tumours of low malignant potential with no stromal invasion

C. Parous women have a reduced risk of developing borderline tumours when compared with nulliparous women
D. Lactation is found to be protective
E. Oral contraceptive use is protective in the development of borderline ovarian tumours

12. **The risk factors for recurrence of borderline ovarian tumours as invasive tumours are, except:**
    A. Invasive implants
    B. DNA aneuploidy
    C. Micropapillary tumours
    D. Large size tumours
    E. High-grade tumours

13. **The features of differentiated VIN are:**
    A. Younger age group
    B. Older women
    C. Multifocal lesion
    D. HPV associated
    E. Risk of progression to SCC

14. **Complications of lichen sclerosus are, except:**
    A. Pseudo-clitoral cyst
    B. Chronic pelvic pain
    C. SCC
    D. Dysaesthesia
    E. Dyspareunia

15. **All the following are used to treat lichen sclerosis except:**
    A. Clobetasol
    B. Tacrolimus
    C. Imiquimod
    D. Acitretin
    E. UVA phototherapy

16. **Vulval cancer of any size with or without extension to adjacent perineal structures with three or more positive inguinofemoral lymph node metastasis is classified as FIGO stage:**
    A. Stage II
    B. Stage IIIA
    C. Stage IIIB
    D. Stage IVA
    E. Stage IB

17. **The endometrial cells in cervical samples may be associated with endometrial pathology if:**
    A. The women under 40 years
    B. The sample taken in follicular phase of menstrual cycle
    C. The sample taken after 14th day of menstrual cycle
    D. The women taking tamoxifen
    E. The women has IUCD fitted in

18. **An excisional biopsy of cervix is recommended in all conditions, except:**
    A. When cytology indicates mild or borderline changes, but normal colposcopy
    B. When cytology indicates moderate dyskaryosis
    C. When cytology indicates severe dyskaryosis
    D. When a recognisably atypical transformation zone on colposcopy
    E. When low grade colposcopic change is associated with severe dyskaryosis or worse

19. **The ablative techniques are suitable to treat CIN only when**
    A. The entire transformation is visualised
    B. There is evidence of glandular abnormality
    C. There is evidence of invasive disease
    D. There is major discrepancy between cytology and histology
    E. There is CIN2, CIN3 or cGIN

20. **Annual cervical screening is advised in**
    A. Women who are HIV positive
    B. Women receiving cytotoxic drugs for rheumatological disorders
    C. Women with renal failure requiring dialysis
    D. Women receiving oestrogen antagonists such as tamoxifen
    E. Women taking long-term steroids

21. **Cervical screening in pregnant women should be performed in all situations, except:**
    A. For routine recall
    B. Who had previous abnormal test
    C. First follow up cytology or colposcopy after treatment for cGIN
    D. First follow up after treatment for CIN2/3
    E. First follow up after treatment for CIN2/3 with uncertain margin status

22. **Unscheduled cervical screening is not justified in the following situations except:**
    A. In women starting to take an oral contraceptive
    B. In women with genital warts
    C. In women with vaginal discharge
    D. In women with pelvic infection
    E. In women who missed previous routine screening interval

23. **The following are the characteristics of type II endometrial carcinoma, except:**
    A. Associated with unopposed oestrogen exposure
    B. Seen in postmenopausal age group
    C. Usually present with deep myometrial invasion
    D. Histologic subtype of serous and clear cell carcinomas
    E. Precursor lesion is endometrial intraepithelial lesion

ANSWERS

1. **(E) HPV vaccine is an inactivated vaccine but not recommended in pregnancy**

   Gardasil is quadrivalent vaccine against HPV6, 11, 16 and 18 introduced in UK in 2012. Both bivalent and quadrivalent vaccines are efficacious in preventing HPV infection. Gardasil is given two dose regimen but in girls who are immunocompromised three dosed should be considered. HPV vaccine is not live vaccine but as matter of precaution it is not recommended in pregnancy. (*Vaccination against cervical cancer scientific impact paper number 9, RCOG.org*).

2. **(B) Alcohol**

   The most important cause for the development of cervical intraepithelial neoplasia (CIN) and cervical cancer is persistent high-risk HPV infection. Several co-factors increase the incidence of invasive cervical cancers such as smoking, increasing number of full term pregnancies, HIV infection, immunocompromised status and contraceptive pill (*Vaccination against cervical cancer scientific impact paper number 9, RCOG.org*).

3. **(C) Perinatal mortality**

   The women with ovarian cancer present with advanced disease. The 5 year survival rate for advanced ovarian cancer between 2005 and 2009 was 43%. (*Targeted therapies for management of ovarian cancer scientific impact paper number 12, RCOG.org*).

4. **(C) If the excision loop was more than 10 mm**

   Cold-knife, laser conisation and LLETZ were all significantly associated with increased risk of preterm birth and low birthweight, while no statistically significant difference was found in perinatal mortality. Cold-knife conisation was also found to be associated with an increased rate of caesarean section. LLETZ is associated with PPROM. (*Obstetric Impact of Treatment for CIN, scientific impact paper number 21, RCOG.org*).

5. **(B) 20–30%**

   The most important known for the development of cervical intraepithelial neoplasia (CIN) and cervical cancer is persistent high-risk HPV infection. Several co-factors increase the incidence of invasive cervical cancers such as smoking, increasing number of full term pregnancies, HIV infection, immunocompromised status and contraceptive pill. (*Vaccination against cervical cancer scientific impact paper number 9, RCOG.org*).

Gynaeoncology

6. **(E) Triple X syndrome**

   Two large meta-analyses concluded that the laser ablation does not affect the obstetric outcomes. (*Obstetric Impact of Treatment for CIN: scientific impact paper number 21, RCOG.org*).

7. **(E) Less than 35 years**

   Approximately 5% of endometrial carcinomas and 20% of epithelial ovarian carcinomas are hereditary. The autosomal dominant disorders, hereditary breast and ovarian cancer (HBOC) and Lynch syndrome (formerly referred to as hereditary nonpolyposis colorectal carcinoma, HNPCC) underlie the majority of this inherited susceptibility. However, rare syndromes such as Cowden, Peutz-Jeghers and Li-Fraumeni can also manifest with gynaecological malignancies. (*Management of women with a genetic predisposition to gynaecological cancers, scientific impact paper number 9, RCOG.org*).

8. **(D) 10–15%**

   In *BRCA1* mutation carriers, the risk may decrease by as much as 56% and for women with a *BRCA2* mutation by up to 46%, with the risk reduction being greatest if surgery is performed before 40 years of age. (*Management of women with a genetic predisposition to gynaecological cancers, scientific impact paper number 9, RCOG.org*).

9. **(B) Neoadjuvant chemotherapy and loop excision in stage I cervical cancer**

   Studies have reported an 80–96% decrease in ovarian cancer risk in *BRCA1* and *BRCA2* mutation carriers who underwent RRBSO. However, there remains a residual 1–6% risk of primary peritoneal cancer that appears to persist for up to 20 years after oophorectomy (*Management of women with a genetic predisposition to gynaecological cancers, scientific impact paper number 9, RCOG.org*).

10. **(A) Minimal access surgery preferred to open laparotomy**

    RVT is considered as a safe option in early adenocarcinoma of cervix as the position of the tumour is important than the histology. Tumours more than 2 cm have higher recurrence rate hence RVT is restricted tumours less than 2 cm. If irradiation of the pelvis becomes essential in the management of cervical cancer in the presence of the pelvic nodal metastasis or parametrial invasion, ovarian transposition may be considered. (*Fertility sparing treatment in Gynaecological cancers; SIP 35, RCOG.org*).

11. **(D) Lactation is found to be protective**

    Laparoscopic surgery is the optimum approach to minimise the postoperative wound complications and encourage early discharge from hospital. Abdominoplasty at open procedures is a time consuming but reduces perioperative morbidity. Primary radiotherapy and progestogens can be considered in women who are unfit for surgery, but recurrence risks are high for both the modalities. (*Endometrial cancer in obese women SIP 32, RCOG.org*).

12. **(E) High-grade tumours**

    Younger women are more likely to have borderline tumours compared with older women. Parity and lactation are found to be protective. However, unlike invasive ovarian cancer, oral contraceptive use is not protective against the development of borderline ovarian tumours. (*Management of borderline ovarian tumours. TOG: volume 14; April, 2012*).

13. **(D) HPV associated**

    The risk recurrence is significantly higher in borderline ovarian tumours with invasive implant, DNA aneuploidy, high-grade tumours and micropapillary tumours. (*Management of borderline ovarian tumours. TOG: volume 14; April, 2012*).

14. **(B) Chronic pelvic pain**

    Usual type of VIN is associated with HPV infection similar to CIN in younger age group. It could be multifocal, frequently seen in immunocompromised and associated with smoking whereas differentiated type of VIN is seen older age group associate with lichen sclerosis and lichen planus. Both have similar malignant potential. (*GTG Number 58: Vulval skin disorders management, RCOG.org*).

15. **(B) Tacrolimus**

    All are complications of lichen sclerosis except chronic pelvic pain. Development of squamous cell carcinoma is less than 5%. (*GTG Number 58: Vulval skin disorders management, RCOG.org*).

16. **(C) Stage IIIB**

    Ultra potent topical steroids as clobetasol propionate are the recommended regimen. Other unlicensed treatments are tacrolimus, acitretin (retinoid) and UVA phototherapy. Imiquimod is used for VIN lesions. (*GTG Number 58: Vulval skin disorders management, RCOG.org*)

17. **(C) The sample taken after 14th day of menstrual cycle**

    FIGO staging Vulval cancer, 2009. (*Squamous vulval cancer—an update. TOG: volume 15; October, 2013*).

18. **(C) When cytology indicates severe dyskaryosis**

    Endometrial pathology is suspected if endometrial cells seen in cervical sample in women over 40 years. If the sample taken in secretory phase of the menstrual cycle. Exceptions are when women receiving oral contraceptives, hormone replacement, tamoxifen or are fitted with an IUCD. In women under 40 endometrial cells in cervical sample has no clinical significance. (*Colposcopy and Programme management: NHSCSP; May, 2010*).

19. **(A) The entire transformation is visualised**

    Low-grade dyskaryosis with positive HPV should be referred to colposcopy and if colposcopy or less than CIN 1, women should discharged for routine recall. In all other, managed on basis of "see and treat". Women with severe dyskaryosis on cytology but low-grade changes on colposcopy, should of at least cervical biopsy. (*Colposcopy and Programme Management: NHSCSP; May, 2010 and Screening Protocol Algorithm for HPV Triage and TOC; July, 2014*).

20. **(A) Women who are HIV positive**

    The ablative techniques are suitable only if
    a. The entire transformation zone is visualised (100%)
    b. There is no evidence of glandular abnormality (100%)
    c. There is no evidence of invasive disease (100%)
    d. There is no major discrepancy between cytology and histology.
    (*Colposcopy and Programme Management; NHSCSP; May, 2010*).

21. **(A) For routine recall**

    In pregnant women cervical screening should deferred if it is a routine recall or follow-up after treatment for CIN 1 and not the first follow-up after treatment for cGIN and CIN 2/3. (*Colposcopy and Programme Management: NHSCSP; May, 2010*).

22. **(A) In women starting to take an oral contraceptive**

    Women who are HIV positive should have annual cytology. Women undergoing renal transplantation should have had cervical cytology performed within as a year. Women who had renal transplantation and on immunosuppression treatment should have cervical screening as per national guidelines for non-immunocompromised. Women who are receiving long-term steroids, oestrogen antagonists such as tamoxifen, and long-term cytotoxic drugs for rheumatologic disorders should have regular cytological screening in accordance with national guidelines. (*Colposcopy and Programme Management: NHSCSP; May, 2010*).

23. **(A) Associated with unopposed oestrogen exposure**

    Type II endometrial cancer (uterine papillary serous or clear cell carcinomas) constitute 10–20% of endometrial cancers. They are usually high grade cancers which invade in a similar fashion to ovarian cancer and also by lympho-vascular space invasion. These are aggressive and have worse prognosis. These are not oestrogen-dependent unlike type I cancer (endometroid adenocarcinoma). (*Malignant Disease of Uterus, StratOG*).

CHAPTER 10

Urogynaecology

1. **Techniques proven of value at the time of hysterectomy in preventing vault prolapse are all except:**
   A. McCall culdoplasty
   B. Suturing cardinal and uterosacral ligaments
   C. Sacrospinous fixation at the time of vaginal hysterectomy
   D. Subtotal hysterectomy
   E. None

2. **Abdominal sacrocolpopexy in comparison to sacrospinous fixation has better outcome except:**
   A. Reduced recurrent vault prolapse
   B. Reduced risk of dyspareunia
   C. Reduces postoperative stress urinary incontinence (SUI)
   D. Lower reoperation rate
   E. None

3. **Sacrospinous fixation is more suitable for:**
   A. Young woman
   B. Woman with history of dyspareunia
   C. With short vaginal length
   D. All
   E. None

4. **Choose statement regarding transvaginal mesh that is incorrect:**
   A. Is first-line treatment for post-hysterectomy vaginal prolapse (PHVP)
   B. Woman should be informed of potential mesh complications
   C. It can have long-term effect that can be difficult to treat
   D. Woman should be fully informed of permanent value of the mesh
   E. All are correct

5. **PHVP is reported in what percentage of woman after a hysterectomy performed for prolapse:**
   A. 1–2%
   B. 5–7%
   C. 10–12%
   D. 15–20%
   E. 25%

6. **PHVP is seen in what percentage of woman who have undergone hysterectomy for other benign diseases:**
   A. <1%
   B. 1–2%
   C. 5%
   D. 8%
   E. 10%
7. **NICE recommends posterior tibial nerve stimulation (PTNS) as a treatment modality only after the below has failed:**
   A. After MDT input
   B. Conservative management has failed
   C. Declines botulinum toxin A
   D. Declines percutaneous sacral nerve stimulation
   E. All of the above
8. **Mirabegron is a:**
   A. Selective beta 1 agonist
   B. Selective beta 2 agonist
   C. Selective beta 3 agonist
   D. Selective alpha agonist
   E. None
9. **NICE recommends offer invasive therapy for overactive bladder (OAB):**
   A. After MDT review
   B. After confirmed urodynamics (UDS) diagnosis
   C. After conservative management fails
   D. After failure of one or more pharmacological agent has failed
   E. All
10. **All women presenting with symptoms of urinary incontinence (UI) should be:**
    A. Offered urine dip
    B. Offered UDS
    C. Offered bladder scan and cystoscopy
    D. Offered antibiotics
    E. All of the above
11. **Woman with following symptoms should be urgently referred to secondary care, except:**
    A. Recurrent UTI
    B. Microscopic haematuria in woman aged 35 years or more
    C. Visible haematuria
    D. Suspected malignant mass arising from urinary tract
    E. None
12. **Indicators for use of long-term indwelling urethral catheter for woman with UI are all except:**
    A. Distress caused by bed and clothing change
    B. Pressure ulcers or irritation from urinary incontinence
    C. Chronic urinary retention in women who are unable to manage to self catheterise
    D. Express preference for this form of management
    E. None

13. **The following drug is useful for nocturia:**
    A. Oxybutynin
    B. Mirabegron
    C. Amitriptyline
    D. Desmopressin
    E. Duloxetine

14. **A UDS shows normal capacity but gradual rise in pressure with bladder filling. This signifies:**
    A. Stress incontinence
    B. Urge incontinence
    C. Voiding dysfunction
    D. Urinary tract infection
    E. Reduced compliance

15. **A UDS shows pressure more than 50 mm Hg and reduced flow rate. Finding correlate most likely with:**
    A. Stress incontinence
    B. Overactive bladder
    C. Voiding dysfunction
    D. Reduced capacity with outflow obstruction
    E. Reduced compliance

16. **Mesh exposure rate:**
    A. 0–1%
    B. 3–5%
    C. 7–8%
    D. 15–20%
    E. 30%

17. **Incorrect statement regarding duloxetine is:**
    A. Is a selective serotonin reuptake inhibitor (SSRI)
    B. Has a role in the treatment for stress incontinence
    C. Side effects of duloxetine are dry mouth, insomnia and suicidal ideation
    D. They are mainly used as antidepressant and for neuropathic pain
    E. Acute angle glaucoma is a contraindication for its use

18. **Mesh erosion usually presents with following symptoms except:**
    A. Pain in back and buttocks
    B. Excessive vaginal discharge
    C. Recurrent UTI
    D. Continuous loss of urine per vagina, unrelated to activity
    E. ALL

19. **Statement that is untrue regarding bladder injury:**
    A. Thermal injury can present in 10–14 days postoperatively
    B. Bladder repair should be sutured in 1 or 2 layers using 2-0 or 3-0 absorbable sutures
    C. Bladder repair should be water tight and tension free
    D. The most common site of injury to the bladder is in the midline, above the inter-ureteric bar
    E. All are correct

20. **Incidence of ureteric injury for a malignant pelvic condition is around:**
    A. 1–2% B. 4–5%
    C. 15% D. 25–30%
    E. 50%

21. **Sacrospinous ligament fixation can be associated with injury to:**
    A. Femoral nerve
    B. Obturator nerve
    C. Genitofemoral nerve
    D. Pudendal nerve
    E. Lateral cutaneous nerve

22. **Transobturator tapes (TOT) can be associated with injury to:**
    A. Obturator nerve
    B. Sciatic nerve
    C. Common peroneal nerve
    D. Genitofemoral nerve
    E. Iliohypogastric

23. **Mesh of choice for Gynaecological surgery:**
    A. Type 1 monofilament polypropylene
    B. Biological mesh
    C. Type 111 non-knitted, non-woven multifilament mesh
    D. Combined mesh
    E. Non-absorbable synthetic mesh

24. **Persistence of urinary incontinence following postpartum is seen in about:**
    A. 1% B. 5%
    C. 15% D. 25%
    E. 50%

25. **Indications for urodynamics testing are all except:**
    A. Identify or rule out the factors contributing to the incontinence
    B. Predict the outcome of intervention
    C. Confirm the effects of treatment
    D. Identify the reasons for failure of previous treatment for incontinence
    E. All are true

26. **Most common type of injury to ureter is:**
    A. Complete transection
    B. Ligation
    C. Excision
    D. Crushing
    E. Partial transection

ANSWERS

1. **(D) Subtotal hysterectomy**

   RCOG GTG Number 46.

   McCall culdoplasty at the time of vaginal hysterectomy is a recommended measure to prevent enterocele formation. The technique involves approximating the uterosacral ligaments using continuous sutures, so as to obliterate the peritoneum of the posterior cul-de-sac as high as possible.

   Suturing the cardinal and uterosacral ligaments to the vaginal cuff at the time of hysterectomy is a recommended measure to avoid vault prolapse.

   Sacrospinous fixation at the time of vaginal hysterectomy is recommended when the vault descends to the introitus during closure.

   Abdominal sacrocolpopexy was associated with significantly longer operating time, slower return to normal activity and higher cost. There was no significant difference in terms of objective and subjective success, urinary, bowel or sexual dysfunction or quality of life. Complications were rare but included: sacrocolpopexy: blood transfusion, bladder injury, mesh rejection, incisional hernia and wound infection. Sacrospinous fixation is associated with blood transfusion, bladder injury, rectovaginal haematoma, and vaginal pain.

2. **(D) Lower reoperation rate**

   RCOG GTG Number 46.

   Abdominal sacrocolpopexy and sacrospinous fixation should be considered in terms of their relative benefits and risks. Abdominal sacrocolpopexy is an effective operation for post-hysterectomy vaginal vault prolapse. In comparison, sacrospinous fixation may have a higher failure rate but has lower postoperative morbidity.

3. **(E) None**

   RCOG GTG Number 46.

4. **(A) Is first-line treatment for post-hysterectomy vaginal prolapse (PHVP)**

   Management of vault prolapse. TOG: volume 15; July, 2013.

   Role of synthetic mesh in the treatment of pelvic organ prolapse. TOG: volume 11; July, 2009.

   Management of vault prolapse. TOG: volume 16; January, 2013.

5. **(C) 10–12%**

   Management of vault prolapse. TOG: volume 15; July, 2013.

   Role of synthetic mesh in the treatment of pelvic organ prolapse. TOG: volume 11; July, 2009.

   Management of vault prolapse. TOG: volume 16; January, 2013.

6. **(B) 1–2%**

   Management of vault prolapse. TOG: volume 15; July, 2013.

   Role of synthetic mesh in the treatment of pelvic organ prolapse. TOG: volume 11; July, 2009.

   Management of vault prolapse. TOG: volume 16; January, 2013.

7. **(E) All of the above**

   NICE guidelines on: The management of urinary incontinence in women

   Offer percutaneous sacral nerve stimulation to women after MDT review if: their OAB has not responded to conservative management including drugs, and they are unable to perform clean intermittent catheterisation. Consider percutaneous sacral nerve stimulation after MDT review if a woman's OAB has not responded to conservative management (including drugs) and botulinum toxin A.

   Discuss the long-term implications of percutaneous sacral nerve stimulation with women including:
   - The need for test stimulation and probability of the test's success
   - The risk of failure
   - The long-term commitment
   - The need for surgical revision
   - The adverse effects.

8. **(C) Selective beta 3 agonist**

   NICE guidelines on: The management of urinary incontinence in women.

9. **(A) After MDT review**

   NICE guidelines on: The management of urinary incontinence in women

   Offer invasive therapy for OAB and/or SUI symptoms only after an MDT review.

10. **(A) Offered urine dip**

    NICE guidelines on: The management of urinary incontinence in women.

    Offer invasive therapy for OAB and/or SUI symptoms only after an MDT review.

11. **(B) Microscopic haematuria in woman aged 35 years or more**

    NICE guidelines on: The management of urinary incontinence in women.
    Urgently refer women with UI who have any of the following:
    - Microscopic haematuria in women aged 50 years and older visible haematuria
    - Recurrent or persisting UTI associated with haematuria in women aged 40 years and older
    - Suspected malignant mass arising from the urinary tract.

12. **(C) Chronic urinary retention in women who are unable to manage to self catheterise**

    NICE guidelines on: The management of urinary incontinence in women.

    Careful consideration should be given to the impact of long-term indwelling urethral catheterization. Practicalities, benefits and risks should be discussed with the patient or, if appropriate, her carer. Indications for the use of long-term indwelling urethral catheters for women with UI include: chronic urinary retention in women who are unable to manage intermittent self-catheterisation skin wounds, pressure ulcers or irritations that are being contaminated by urine distress or disruption caused by bed and clothing changes where a woman expresses a preference for this form of management.

    Indwelling suprapubic catheters should be considered as an alternative to long-term urethral catheters.

13. **(E) Duloxetine**

    NICE guidelines on: The management of urinary incontinence in women.

    The use of desmopressin may be considered specifically to reduce nocturia in women with UI or OAB who find it a troublesome symptom. Use particular caution in women with cystic fibrosis and avoid in those over 65 years with cardiovascular disease or hypertension.

14. **(E) Reduced compliance**

    NICE guidelines on: The management of urinary incontinence in women. Basics of Urodynamics.

15. **(D) Reduced capacity with outflow obstruction**

    NICE guidelines on: The management of urinary incontinence in women. Basics of urodynamics

16. **(C) 7–8%**

    Mesh erosion may present with varied symptoms, constant infections, clear slimy discharge, bleeding, pain in the lower back and buttocks, internal and external abscess and itching. Another symptom on mesh erosion is the dragging feeling, as if something is stuck like a large tampon and feels very abrasive, the medical world seems to use the term—a cheese grater. Other symptoms they may present with is very difficult to sit and walk and also very uncomfortable while having sex.

    Erosion is due to shrinkage of the mesh, recent studies have shown that mesh shrinks 10% each year with 85% contracture at 8 years. It has been shown 10% women with mesh go back to theatre for removal/trimming of the mesh.

17. **(A) Is a selective serotonin reuptake inhibitor (SSRI)**

    Duloxetine is a serotonin-norepinephrine reuptake inhibitor (SNRI). It is widely used for major depressive disorder, generalized anxiety disorder, neuropathic pain specially cancer related and fibromyalgia. NICE does not recommend as 1st or 2nd line treatment for stress incontinence but it can be offered as second-line for stress incontinence when other methods have failed or not suitable and is patient's choice over surgery. It is associated with nausea, dizziness, somnolence, insomnia, dry mouth, headache and sexual dysfunction. It should be used with caution due to known side effect of suicidal ideation. Several studies have shown that it can decrease the incontinence episode frequency up to 50% but discontinuation rates are quite high due to its side effects and this is very much dose related.

18. **(D) Continuous loss of urine per vagina, unrelated to activity**

    Mesh erosion may present with varied symptoms, constant infections, clear slimy discharge, bleeding, pain in the lower back and buttocks, internal and external abscess and itching. Another symptom on mesh erosion is the dragging feeling, as if something is stuck like a large tampon and feels very abrasive, the medical world seems to use the term—a cheese grater. Other symptoms they may present with is very difficult to sit and walk and also very uncomfortable while having sex. Erosion is due to shrinkage of the mesh, recent studies have shown that mesh shrinks 10% each year with 85% contracture at 8 years. It has been shown 10% women with mesh go back to theatre for removal/trimming of the mesh.

19. **(E) All are correct**

20. **(D) 25–30%**

    Incidence of ureteric injury following benign gynaecology surgery is around 2.5–4%, whereas the incidence is highly increased for malignant gynaecology surgery and the incidence is as high as 30%. The injury occurs most frequently in the lower third of the ureter (51%), followed by the upper third (30%) and the middle third (19%). Most studies show the most common site of injury to be lateral to the ureteric vessels and at the ovarian fossa.

21. **(D) Pudendal nerve**

    Refer to TOG 2014 Number 1.

    The patient will report postoperative gluteal, perineal and vulval pain, which worsen in the seated position. It can be associated with sexual dysfunction.

22. **(A) Obturator nerve**

    Refer to TOG 2014 Number 1.

    Obturator neuropathy will present with sensory loss in the upper medial thigh and motor weakness in the hip adductors.

23. **(A) Type 1 monofilament polypropylene**

    Refer to TOG 2009, Volume 11, Issue 3.

    The mechanical properties of the synthetic mesh depend on the structure of the fabric and the thread. The tensile strength of permanent synthetic mesh is highly variable, depending on fibre type, weight: area ratio and weave. To increase versatility, materials can be structured from monofilament or multifilament fibres, which can be twisted, coated, braided or double-braided.

24. **(D) 25%**

    Refer to TOG 2012,Volume 14, Issue 3.

    The management of urogynaecological problems in pregnancy and the early postpartum period. Urinary tract infection (UTI) is the most common medical complication of pregnancy. The incidence of asymptomatic bacteriuria during pregnancy is 2–5% and if not treated, up to 20% of women will develop a lower UTI. The overall incidence of UTI in pregnancy is 8%. Women should be counselled that pregnancy and delivery may have a deleterious effect on the outcome of previous surgery and that elective caesarean section may be only partially protective. MacArthur et al. found that delivery exclusively by caesarean section was associated with less persistent urinary incontinence compared with those delivered by caesarean section in addition to vaginal delivery; however, the prevalence of persistent symptoms is still high (14%).

25. **(E) All are true**

    Refer to TOG 2006, Volume 8, and Issue 2.

26. **(A) Complete transection**

    The incidences of different forms of injury are complete transection 61%, excision 29%, ligation 7%, and partial transection 3%. Other forms of injury are by avascular necrosis following extensive dissection and kinking as well.

CHAPTER 11

Miscellaneous Topics

1. Which of the above is a strong tool for assessing doctor-patient relationship?
   A. CBD
   B. Mini-CEX
   C. DOPS
   D. OSAT
   E. ALL
2. Which is not a component of 5 steps of "The 1-minute Preceptor"?
   A. Commitment
   B. Positive reinforcement
   C. Judgement
   D. Application
   E. Correction of mistakes
3. The below method is good method of teaching in trainees in relatively early stage of teaching:
   A. Schema refinement
   B. Brainstorming
   C. Snowballing
   D. Lectures
   E. None
4. Average retention rate with lectures is:
   A. 5%
   B. 25%
   C. 50%
   D. 75%
   E. 100%
5. What does not apply for an advance directive?
   A. Can be made by anyone aged more than 18 years
   B. Must be writing if—sustaining treatment is being refused
   C. Oral advance directive are never binding
   D. Failure to recognize an AD may give rise to civil wrong of trespass. (legal action)
   E. Refusal of basic nursing cannot be made in AD
6. What is true regarding mental capacity?
   A. Is age related, never task oriented
   B. Can be established by reference to a person's previous behaviour
   C. Patient who are only able to retain information for a short period are regarded as lacking capacity
   D. Capacity is not fixed in time and hence can change depending on circumstances
   E. None

7. **The main challenge faced by clinical trials/studies is:**
   A. Lower than expected rates of recruitment
   B. Difficulty in collaborating with other centre
   C. Funding
   D. Getting ethical approval
   E. None

8. **Only ---- of randomized trials in UK are able to meet the recruitment targets.**
   A. One-third
   B. One-fourth
   C. Half
   D. Three-quarter
   E. One-tenth

9. **Failure to recruit to the target number in a clinical trial can lead to:**
   A. Underpowered study
   B. Premature closure of the trial
   C. Increased risk of reporting falsely that the observed clinically relevant differences are not significant
   D. All
   E. None

10. **A woman with pathological CTG declines caesarean section in spite of understanding risk of foetal death is**
    A. Autonomy
    B. Virtual
    C. Veracity
    D. Paternalism
    E. Therapeutic privilege

11. **Agreeing to insert Mirena in a mentally handicapped girl suffering from severe menorrhagia is**
    A. Autonomy
    B. Beneficence
    C. Justice
    D. Utilitarianism
    E. Munificence

12. **Early warning signs of a trainee in difficulty are all except:**
    A. Disappearing act
    B. Ward rage
    C. Rigidity
    D. Career progression
    E. Low work rate

13. **Multisource feedback looks into following except:**
    A. Reliability
    B. Record keeping
    C. Team working
    D. Leadership
    E. All

14. **Regarding workplace-based assessment, the correct statement is:**
    A. WPBA uses Millers pyramid to assess competency
    B. WPBA tools are CBD, mini-CEX, OSAT
    C. RCOG recommends only consultants should act as assessor in WPBA encounters
    D. Reflection on a task and developing an insight is regarded as hall mark of adult learning and is requirement for GMC (General medical council) revalidation.
    E. None

15. **Which is incorrect statement regarding analgesia in labour?**
    A. First stage of labour pain is transmitted via T10–L1 nerves
    B. Second stage labour pain is transmitted via S2–S4 nerve roots
    C. There is strong evidence to prove acupuncture can reduce labour pain
    D. Sterile water injection in painful area can reduce pain in labour
    E. Immersion in water reduces labour pain
16. **Studies show birthing ball and birthing positions are associated with:**
    A. Reduction in labour pain
    B. Less use of analgesics
    C. Shorter first stage of labour
    D. Reduces caesarean section
    E. All
17. **Correct statement regarding nitrous oxide is:**
    A. Can cause delay in second stage
    B. Causes respiratory depression
    C. Prolonged N_2O exposure in health workers has been linked to decrease in fertility and preterm birth
    D. Several studies have supported its use as an effective analgesic for labour pain
    E. None
18. **Choose the incorrect statement:**
    A. Neonates may take up to 6 hours to eliminate pethidine from its system
    B. Diamorphine can prolong delivery
    C. Diamorphine is associated with significant increase in neonatal adverse outcome
    D. Diamorphine gives better analgesia than pethidine
    E. None
19. **Incorrect statement regarding patient-controlled analgesia (PCA):**
    A. Remifentanil is most commonly used drug for PCA
    B. It can be associated with respiratory depression and low oxygen saturation
    C. Common adverse effect of remifentanil is pruritus', nausea and vomiting
    D. There can be potential tolerance after some time, resulting in reduction in its effectiveness
    E. All are correct
20. **Epidural can be associated with:**
    A. Permanent nerve injury and paraplegia
    B. Prolonged second stage of labour
    C. Most common side effect of combined spinal and epidural (CSE) is nausea and vomiting
    D. CEFM should be performed for 30 minutes during establishment of epidural and after bolus of more than 10 mL
    E. All are correct statement

21. **Incidence of breast cancer in pregnancy:**
    A. 1:1,000
    B. 1:2,000
    C. 1:3,000
    D. 1:5,000
    E. 1:10,000

22. **What percentage of women in UK are offered invasive prenatal diagnostic tests?**
    A. 0.5%
    B. 1%
    C. 5%
    D. 10%
    E. 15%

23. **Following favour occipito-posterior position**
    A. Gynaecoid pelvis
    B. Anthropoid pelvis
    C. Platypelloid pelvis
    D. Anthropoid and Android pelvis
    E. Unrelated

24. **Which of the statements regarding domestic abuse are false?**
    A. 20% of women in England and Wales have suffered DA at some point of time
    B. More than 40% cases first start during pregnancy
    C. 40–60% of women of DA are abused during pregnancy
    D. More than 14% of maternal deaths occur in women who have informed their health professionals about their abusive relationship
    E. More than 50% of known DA cases, children were also abused

25. **Contraindications to low molecular weight heparin (LMWH)**
    A. Women with active bleeding
    B. Women with bleeding diathesis
    C. Women with thrombocytosis
    D. Acute stroke in last 4 weeks
    E. Severe liver disease

26. **Lifetime increase in risk of breast cancer with CTPA**
    A. 0.1%
    B. 1%
    C. 10%
    D. 13%
    E. 25%

27. **Epidural catheter should not be removed within ---------hours of recent LMWH injection.**
    A. 4 hours
    B. 8 hours
    C. 12 hours
    D. 24 hours

28. **Background risk of having major congenital anomaly is seen in:**
    A. 1%
    B. 2–3%
    C. 5–7%
    D. 10%
    E. 0.1%

29. **A 23-year-old gives birth to baby with Down's syndrome. In what percentage, translocation accounts for this condition?**
    A. 2–3%
    B. 10%
    C. 80%
    D. 96%
    E. 0.1%

30. **Cystic hygroma is strongly associated with the following condition:**
    A. Down's syndrome
    B. Klinefelter syndrome
    C. Turner's syndrome
    D. Edward syndrome
    E. None

31. **Mickey mouse head appearance is referred to following condition:**
    A. Anencephaly
    B. Down syndrome
    C. Dandy Walker malformation
    D. DiGeorge syndrome
    E. Cri du-chat syndrome

32. **A 22-year-old is seen in pre-pregnancy clinic, she is known to have large VSD. What is the risk of her having a baby with congenital heart disease?**
    A. 1%
    B. 2%
    C. 6%
    D. 10%
    E. 25%

ANSWERS

1. **(B) Mini-CEX**

   Refer to TOG 2010; volume 12 number 4.

   The mini-clinical evaluation exercise (mini-CEX) consists of a consultation between a patient and the learner, which is observed and assessed by the teacher. The mini-CEX is a powerful tool for assessing doctor-patient communication, diagnostic acumen and treatment planning.

2. **(C) Judgement**

   Refer to TOG 2010; volume 12 number 4.

   This is a five-step process that can be carried out in 15 minutes with the purpose of structuring teaching opportunities that arise in the clinical environment.

   The five steps are:
   1. Commitment
   2. Justification
   3. Application
   4. Positive reinforcement
   5. Correction of mistakes

3. **(B) Brainstorming**

   Refer to TOG 2010; volume 12 number 4.

   This is a spontaneous group discussion to produce ideas and ways of solving a problem. The clinical teacher may use this method to promote clinical and critical thinking in trainees who are at a relatively early stage in their career.

4. **(A) 5%**

   Refer to TOG 2010; volume 12 number 4.

   This is an educational talk to an audience and is the teaching method with which most clinicians are comfortable. There are potential drawbacks. Participation by learners is minimal, there is a risk that the lecturer can appear patronizing and ulterior motives may be suspected.

5. **(C) Oral advance directive are never binding**

   Refer to TOG 2010; volume 12 number 1

   Anyone over the age of 18 years can make an advance decision. Below this age, the courts can overrule decisions to refuse life-saving treatment when not in the patient's best interests. An advance decision must be specific to the treatment that is being refused and will only apply when the person lacks capacity. Patients do not have the right to demand a specific treatment; they can only refuse treatment. An order for an advance decision to be valid in relation to life-sustaining treatment the medical circumstances must be specifically mentioned in the directive and comply with Section 25(6) of the Act. Basic or essential nursing care such as basic hygiene, shelter and warmth, moving patients to avoid bedsores, cleanliness and food cannot be refused in any advance decision, since this would be regarded as inhumane.

6. **(D) Capacity is not fixed in time and hence can change depending on circumstances**

    Refer to TOG 2010 volume 12 no 1.

    Anyone in the UK over the age of 18 years is legally defined as an adult. However, the Mental Capacity Act 2005 applies to anyone aged 16 years and above; over this age, there is a presumption of legal capacity unless otherwise established [section 1(2) of the Act] and so any decision (even an unwise one) is protected in law. Capacity is not fixed in time; it is dynamic and can thus wax and wane, particularly during periods of fluctuating consciousness and pain.

7. **(A) Lower than expected rates of recruitment**

    Refer to TOG 2015 volume 17 Issue 1.

    One of the main challenges faced by clinical studies, both nationally and internationally, is the lower than expected rates of recruitment. One of the keys to successful recruitment is collaboration and collective effort. Multicentre involvement has an extraordinarily positive impact on recruitment in clinical trials.

8. **(A) One-third**

    Refer to TOG 2015; volume 17 Issue 1.

    Only a third of the randomized trials in the UK meet their recruitment targets and more than half need to be extended. Many studies face premature closure due to futile recruitment and recruitment of smaller sample size than originally planned leads to an underpowered study and risk of reporting falsely that the observed clinically relevant differences are not significant.

9. **(D) All**

    Refer to TOG; 2015; volume 17 Issue 1.

10. **(A) Autonomy**

    Refer to TOG 2010; volume 12 issue 1.

    This is woman's autonomy; similar situation is described when a woman declines blood or blood products.

    In such situation, there is conflict between beneficence and woman's autonomy.

    - Virtual—means almost or nearly as described
    - Veracity—truthfulness
    - Munificence—act of generosity

- Paternalism—practice of treating/governing people in a fatherly manner or providing for their needs without giving them the rights.

11. **(B) Beneficence**

    Refer to TOG 2010; volume 12 issue 1.

12. **(D) Career progression**

    Refer to TOG 2011; Issue 4.

    The features of a trainee in trouble are disappearing act, low work rate, ward rage, rigidity, bypass syndrome, career problems, and insight failure.

13. **(C) Team working**

    Refer to TOG 2011; Issue 4.

    Multisource feedback looks into communication, record keeping, teamwork, leadership, reliability, etc.

14. **(C) RCOG recommends only consultants should act as assessor in WPBA encounters**

    Refer to TOG 2014; volume 16.

15. **(C) There is strong evidence to prove acupuncture can reduce labour pain**

    Refer to TOG 2015; volume 17 Issue 3.

16. **(E) All**

    Refer to TOG 2015; volume 17 Issue 3.

    One RCT demonstrates birthing balls and position can cause reduction in labour pain by 30–40%. It reduces epidural requirement, shorter first stage of labour and fewer caesarean sections. Upright positions also appear to shorten the second stage of labour, reduces instrumental delivery rates and episiotomies but increase blood loss.

17. **(C) Prolonged N_2O exposure in health workers has been linked to decrease in fertility and preterm birth**

    Refer to TOG 2015; volume 17 Issue 3.

    Nitrous oxide is unlikely to affect the labour process. While it crosses the placenta readily, nitrous oxide does not affect the foetal heart rate or respiratory rate in the newborn. Common adverse effects include lightheadedness, nausea, vomiting and less commonly, hallucination, hyperventilation and tetany. In trials comparing nitrous oxide with a placebo, pain scores are lower in women in the nitrous oxide group.

18. **(C) Diamorphine is associated with significant increase in neonatal adverse outcome**

    Refer to TOG 2015; volume 17 Issue 3.

    Opioids will often produce a prolonged "sleep phase" pattern on cardiotocography, with reduction in foetal heart rate variability, acceleration and decelerations. A neonate may take up to 6 days to eliminate pethidine from its system, with respiratory depression, hypothermia, poor feeding, altered crying and decreased alertness as recognized adverse effects.

19. **(E) All are correct**

    Refer to TOG 2015; volume 17 Issue 3.

    The most widely used opioid for PCA in UK is remifentanil. Remifentanil is rapidly acting synthetic opioids, and has a very short half-life of 3 minutes. One-third of labour units in UK offers remifentanil PCA as a form of analgesia. Adverse effects include respiratory depression, nausea, vomiting and pruritus. There is potential tolerance that may occur after just 60 minutes of use resulting in reduction in efficiency.

20. **(C) Most common side effect of combined spinal and epidural (CSE) is nausea and vomiting**

    Refer to TOG 2015; volume 17 Issue 3.

21. **(C) 1:3,000**

    Refer to GTG: Breast cancer and pregnancy.

22. **(C) 5%**

    Refer to RCOG GTG Number 8; June, 2010.

    It is estimated that around 5% of the pregnant population (approximately 30,000 women per annum in the UK) are offered a choice of invasive prenatal diagnostic tests (most commonly amniocentesis or chorionic villus sampling). Amniocentesis is the most common invasive prenatal diagnostic procedure undertaken in the UK. Most amniocenteses are performed to obtain amniotic fluid for karyotyping from 15 weeks. Amniocentesis performed before 15 completed weeks of gestation is referred to as "early amniocentesis". Chorionic villus sampling (CVS) is usually performed between 11 weeks and 13 weeks. Amniocentesis is the most common invasive prenatal diagnostic procedure undertaken in the UK. Most amniocenteses are performed to obtain amniotic fluid for karyotyping from 15 weeks onwards.

23. **(D) Anthropoid and Android Pelvis**

    Refer to Essential of Obstetrics by Arulkumaran

    The shape of the pelvis: Anthropoid and android pelvises are the most common cause of occipito-posterior due to narrow fore-pelvis.

    Right occipito-posterior (ROP) is more common than left occipito-posterior (LOP) because:

    The left oblique diameter is reduced by the presence of sigmoid colon.

    The right oblique diameter is slightly longer than the left one.

    Dextro-rotation of the uterus favours occipito-posterior in right occipito-anterior position.

24. **(B) More than 40% cases first start during pregnancy**

    Refer to 30% of domestic abuse starts in pregnancy. A handbook for health professionals (London).

25. **(C) Women with thrombocytosis**

    Refer to GTG Number 37a.

    Severe thrombocytopenia is a contraindication.

26. **(D) 13%**

    Lifetime risk is increased by 13.6% with CTPA.

    Refer to GTG Number 37a.

27. **(C) 12 hours**

    Refer to GTG Number 37b

28. **(B) 2–3%**

    Refer to BINOCAR registers; July, 2012.

29. **(A) 2–3%**

    The overall incidence of Down syndrome is 1 in 700 live births. The incidence is higher at conception, but 60% of cases are spontaneously aborted and 20% are stillborn. The incidence of Down syndrome increases with maternal age.

    There is a significant risk of congenital heart disease in Down syndrome with 40% of children being affected. Of these, the most common is atrioventricular septal defects (AVSD). Other complications include duodenal atresia, cataracts (2%), epilepsy (10%), acute leukaemia (1%) and early-onset dementia (in 50% by the age of 50 years).

    The majority (96%) of trisomy 21 arises from non-disjunction in meiosis. This arises from the maternal cell line in 85% of cases and from the father in 15% of cases. 2–3% of cases arise from a parental balanced translocation involving chromosome 21 or as a result of a de novo translocation. The final 1% are mosaics.

30. **(C) Turner's syndrome**

    Turner syndrome only affects females, is common at conception but the majority of affected foetuses miscarry to give an incidence at birth of approximately 1:2,500. The condition can be suspected antenatally in the second trimester with the finding of oedema, which can be generalised (hydrops) or localised to the back of the foetal neck (cystic hygroma). The most common finding on chromosome analysis is 45, XO. The recurrence risk is not increased above the general population.

    Clinical features include a wide carrying angle at the elbow, neck webbing, short stature, peripheral lymphoedema (40%), primary ovarian failure (due to streak gonads) and a low hairline. There is associated congenital heart disease in up to 20% of cases—typically coarctation of the aorta and atrial septal defect.

31. **(A) Anencephaly**

    Refer to Chatzipapas IK, Whitlow BJ, Economides DL. The 'Mickey Mouse' sign and the diagnosis of anencephaly in early pregnancy. Ultrasound Obstet Gynecol. 1999;13(3):196-9.

    In medical imaging literature, a Mickey Mouse appearance has been given to imaging features that depict that of a Mickey Mouse when viewed from the front. It has been described with.
    - Anencephaly
    - Progressive supranuclear palsy.

32. **(C) 6%**

    In the general population, about 1% of all children are born with congenital heart disease. However, the risk increases when either parent has CHD, or when another sibling was born with CHD. Most congenital heart defects result from problems early in the child's heart development, the cause of which is unknown. However, certain environmental and genetic risk factors may play a role. They include: rubella, diabetes, medication, alcohol, smoking, hereditary.

Appendices

Practice Question Paper 1

1. **What percentage of couples need complex treatment for subfertility?**
   - A. 0.1%
   - B. 1%
   - C. 5%
   - D. 8%
   - E. 20%

2. **End target set by HFEA for multiple pregnancy rates with in vitro fertilization (IVF):**
   - A. 5%
   - B. 10%
   - C. 15%
   - D. 20%
   - E. 25%

3. **IVF accounts for _____ percentage of birth in UK.**
   - A. 0.1%
   - B. 1%
   - C. 3–5%
   - D. 10–12%
   - E. 15%

4. **Properties of clomiphene citrate are following except:**
   - A. Anti-oestrogen
   - B. Acts on hypothalamus
   - C. Ovulation rate is 75%
   - D. Pregnancy rate 40%
   - E. Multiple pregnancy rate 1%

5. **Prognosis of vulval cancer depends on following except:**
   - A. Lymph node metastasis
   - B. Does not depend on histological grading
   - C. Depth of invasion
   - D. Staging
   - E. Age and performance of patient

6. **What contraceptive advice would you recommend a woman with history of breast cancer a year back?**
   - A. Combined hormonal pill
   - B. Progestogen-only pill
   - C. DMPA (depot medroxyprogesterone acetate)
   - D. Copper intrauterine device
   - E. Mirena

7. **During surgery for VIN:**
   A. 1 mm margin should be left in a fresh specimen
   B. 1 cm margin should be left in a fresh specimen
   C. 2 mm margin should be left in a fixed specimen
   D. 5 mm margin should be left in a fixed specimen
   E. 15 mm margin should be left in a fresh specimen

8. **What percentage of women are offered invasive antenatal diagnostic techniques?**
   A. 0.1%
   B. 1%
   C. 5%
   D. 10%
   E. None

9. **Severe sepsis with septic shock is associated with mortality in:**
   A. 10%
   B. 20%
   C. 40%
   D. 60%
   E. 80%

10. **What percentage of women labour before the scheduled ERCS?**
    A. 1%
    B. 5%
    C. 10%
    D. 20%
    E. 25%.

11. **What percentage of women are present with recurrent reduced foetal movements?**
    A. 1–2%
    B. 3–5%
    C. 8–10%
    D. 12–15%
    E. None.

12. **Number of cases associated with severe haemorrhage every year in UK:**
    A. 1,000
    B. 2,000
    C. 4,000
    D. 5,000
    E. 10,000

13. **Each year of breastfeeding reduces breast cancer by:**
    A. 1%
    B. 4%
    C. 10%
    D. 15%
    E. 25%

14. **Spontaneous version after 36 weeks of gestation is seen in:**
    A. 1%
    B. 5%
    C. 8%
    D. 15%
    E. 25%

15. **Approximate number of girls at risk of female genital mutilation (FGM) in UK:**
    A. 1,000
    B. 10,000
    C. 20,000
    D. 80,000
    E. 1,00,000

16. **Shoulder dystocia can be associated with permanent disability in:**
    A. 0.1% B. 1%
    C. 5% D. 10%
    E. 25%

17. **Risk of recurrence of a third degree tear is:**
    A. 1–2% B. 4–6%
    C. 10–12% D. 15–20%
    E. None

18. **Very preterm labour accounts for:**
    A. 0.1% B. 1–2%
    C. 5% D. 8–10%
    E. 12%

19. **Following statement regarding uterine artery embolization (UAE) are true except:**
    A. About a third of woman would require a second intervention by 5 years
    B. Woman with symptomatic fibroid, UAE should be considered as one of the treatment options alongside surgical, medical and conservative management
    C. The evidence of fertility and pregnancy outcomes after UAE is good
    D. Patient for UAE should be selected and assessed by MDT
    E. The outcomes after UAE in terms of symptom control are identical to those for hysterectomy

20. **Premature ovarian failure after UAE is seen in:**
    A. 0.1% B. 1–2%
    C. 5% D. 10%
    E. 15%

21. **Contraindications to UAE are all except:**
    A. Recent pelvic infection
    B. Serious doubt as to the diagnosis
    C. Asymptomatic fibroids
    D. Patient declines hysterectomy under any circumstance
    E. None

22. **Post-treatment infection following UAE is seen in:**
    A. 0.1% B. 1–2%
    C. 5% D. 10%
    E. 15%

23. **Incidence of ectopic pregnancy in UK:**
    A. 1 per 1,000 pregnancies B. 11 per 1,000 pregnancies
    C. 20 per 1,000 pregnancies D. 5 per 100 pregnancies.
    E. None

24. **Maternal mortality associated with ectopic pregnancy is estimated as:**
    A. 0.1 per 1,000 ectopic pregnancies
    B. 0.2 per 1,000 ectopic pregnancies
    C. 1 per 1,000 ectopic pregnancies
    D. 1 per 100 ectopic pregnancies
    E. None

25. **NICE recommends expectant management for 7–14 days as first-line for confirmed missed miscarriage, except:**
    A. The woman is at increased risk of haemorrhage
    B. Had previous traumatic experience
    C. There is evidence of infection
    D. Recurrent miscarriage
    E. None

26. **NICE recommends early pregnancy unit should accept self-referrals from following except:**
    A. Woman who had recurrent miscarriage
    B. Previous ectopic pregnancy
    C. Previous molar pregnancy
    D. Women with bleeding
    E. None

27. **Indications for medical management for ectopic pregnancy are all except:**
    A. No significant pain
    B. Haemodynamically stable
    C. Serum beta hCG more than 1,500 IU/L
    D. Adnexal mass less than 35 mm
    E. None

28. **NICE recommends surgery should be offered as first-line of treatment in a woman with confirmed ectopic except:**
    A. Significant pain
    B. Foetal heart present
    C. Beta hCG greater than 5,000 IU/L
    D. Haemodynamically stable
    E. None

29. **There is a risk of need for further treatment in a woman who have undergone salpingotomy:**
    A. 1 in 2
    B. 1 in 4
    C. 1 in 5
    D. 1 in 10
    E. 1 in 100

30. **Diagnosis of endometriosis is made based on:**
    A. Clinical history
    B. Ultrasound scan (USS)
    C. Laparoscopy
    D. Clinical history, USS, laparoscopy and biopsy
    E. Clinical history, USS, laparoscopy and biopsy and immunological markers

31. **Which statement regarding male infertility is untrue?**
    A. In about 50% of men with poor semen quality, no cause will be identified
    B. More than 35 years reduces the chance of achieving a pregnancy by one-tenth as compared with paternal age of less than 25 years
    C. There is an elevated LH and FSH level with normal testosterone in testicular failure
    D. Varicocele is found in 10–12% of men with normal semen
    E. Varicocele is more commonly found on left side

32. **Hypogonadotrophic hypogonadism accounts for:**
    A. <1%
    B. 4–5%
    C. 10%
    D. 15%
    E. 25%

33. **Hormonal levels that are recommended to measure in men with sperm counts of less than 5 million per mL:**
    A. LH and FSH
    B. LH, FSH and testosterone
    C. LH, FSH, testosterone and prolactin
    D. LH, FSH, testosterone, prolactin and testicular biopsy
    E. LH, FSH, testosterone, prolactin and karyotyping.

34. **Micro-deletion in one or more gene of the long arm of the Y chromosome is seen in _____ of men with azoospermia.**
    A. 1%
    B. 5–10%
    C. 10–15%
    D. 25%
    E. >50%

35. **Regarding anti-Mullerian hormone (AMH) statement which is untrue:**
    A. Glycoprotein
    B. In males is expressed by the Sertoli cells of the testes
    C. In females is expressed by granulosa cells of the ovary
    D. AMH is a good indicator of the size of the ovarian antral follicle pool
    E. All are true

ANSWERS

1. **(D)** 8%

   Refer to HFEA 2010

   8% of the population remain sub fertile and require more complex treatment such as assisted conception techniques. Half will have primary subfertility (i.e. no previous pregnancy achieved) and the remainder will have secondary subfertility.

2. **(B) 10%**

   Refer to "Improving outcomes for fertility patients: multiple births 2015 HFEA"

   Historically, the percentage of multiple births as a result of in vitro fertilisation (IVF) treatment has been much higher than natural conceptions, largely because of the trend to transfer two or more embryos to the womb during treatment. In 2008, for example, almost a quarter of births resulting from IVF treatment were of two or more babies. From 2009, following a public consultation, we started setting a maximum multiple birth rate target for clinics to meet. This target started at 24% and was reduced in steps over a period of years to work towards an end goal of reducing the rate to no more than 10% of all live births.

3. **(C) 3-5%**

   Refer to "Fertility treatment in 2010 TRENDS & FIGURES (HFEA)"

   During this time, the proportion of those babies born who were IVF babies has steadily increased. In 1992, 0.3% of all babies were born as a result of IVF treatment; in 2002 this had reached 1.4%. In 2009, nearly 2% of all babies born in the UK were conceived as a result of IVF treatment. The live birth rate after IVF has increased from only 14%, to nearly a quarter by 2009.

4. **(E) Multiple pregnancy rate 1%**

   www.advancedfertility.com

   Side effects of Clomiphene citrate are nausea, vomiting, blurred vision, breast discomfort, stomach discomfort, flushing and ovarian enlargement.

5. **(B) Does not depend on histological grading**

   Refer to TOG 2013

   Vulval cancers account for 3–5% of female genital tract cancers. 90% of tumors are squamous in origin.

6. **(D) Copper intrauterine device**

   Refer to UKMEC for contraceptive use –FSRH

7. **(E) 15 mm margin should be left in a fresh specimen.**

   Refer to RCOG guidelines for the Diagnosis and Management of Vulval cancer May 2014 Surgery to the primary tumour should be radical enough to remove the tumour with adequate margins. The incidence of vulval recurrence has been shown to be related to the measured disease—free surgical margin, as measured in the fixed histopathological specimen. Given the reduction and contraction of tissues following excision and fixation, this equates to at least a 15 mm margin on the fresh surgical specimen. The risk of recurrence increases as the disease—free margins decrease (> 8.0 mm: 0%; < 8.0 mm, 47%). Therefore, wide radical local excision with a minimum margin of 15 mm of disease—free tissue on all margins should be sufficient.

8. **(C) 5%**

   Refer to GTG No. 8 2010

   It is estimated that around 5% of the pregnant population (approximately 30 000 women per annum in the UK) are offered a choice of invasive prenatal diagnostic tests (most commonly amniocentesis or chorionic villus sampling).

9. **(C) 40%**

   Refer to MBRRACE

   There has been significant decrease in the mortality rate from genital tract sepsis in the UK sine 2006-08 when there were 1.13 maternal deaths per 100,000 maternities; the rate of maternal mortality from genital tract sepsis in 2010-12 was 0.5 per 100.000 maternities.

10. **(C) 10%**

    Refer to GTG NO 45 OCTOBER 2015

    As up to 10% of women scheduled for ERCS go into labor before 39 weeks. It is good practice to discuss and document a plan for delivery if labor starts prior to the scheduled date.

11. **(B) 3–5%**

    Refer to GTG No. 57

    When a woman recurrently perceives RFM, her case should be reviewed to exclude predisposing causes, ultrasound assessment should be undertaken as part of investigations. There is association of poor perinatal outcome in women presenting with recurrent RFM.

12. **(C) 4,000**

    Blood loss more than 2000 mL is referred as severe PPH. Hemorrhage is the leading cause of maternal death worldwide accounting for 50% of maternal death in some countries, whereas in UK it accounts for 10% of all direct maternal death.

13. **(B) 4%**

    Refer to GTG No. 12 March 2011

    Fewer than 10% of women diagnosed with breast cancer subsequently become pregnant, Factors that increase the risk of breast cancer are nulliparity, early menarche, increased age at first pregnancy, and carriers of BRCA1 & BRCA2. Transient increase is seen immediately after pregnancy. Factors reducing breast cancer are multiparity, pre-eclampsia, breast-feeding.

    The rate of disease recurrence is highest in the first 3 years after diagnosis.

14. **(C) 8%**

    Refer to GTG No.20a

    Incidence of breech at term is 3–4%. Spontaneous version rate for nulliparous women are approximately 8% after 36weeks but less than 5% after unsuccessful ECV. Spontaneous reversion to breech presentation after successful ECV occurs is less than 5%.

15. **(D) 80,000**

    Refer to GTG No.53 July 2015

    It is estimated by UNICEF that 125 million women worldwide have undergone genital mutilation and that some 2million women undergo some form of genital mutilation annually.

16. **(D) 10%**

    Refer to GTG No. 42 March 2012

    Incidence of shoulder dystocia is between 0.58% and 0.7%. Brachial plexus injury is one of the most important fetal complications of shoulder dystocia, complicating 2.3% to 16% of such deliveries. Most cases of BPI resolve without permanent disability, with fewer than 10% resulting in permanent neurological dysfunction.

17. **(B) 4–6%**

    The overall incidence in UK is 2.9%, with an incidence of 6.1% in primiparous compared with 1.7% in multiparous.

18. **(B) 1–2%**

    Refer to GTG No. 18 February 2011

    Very preterm birth accounts for 1.4% of UK births but 51% of infant deaths. Risk of death or neurosensory disability increases with decreasing gestational age. Preterm birth may have psychological and emotional effects on the family, as well as being costly for health services.

19. **(B) Woman with symptomatic fibroid, UAE should be considered as one of the treatment options alongside surgical, medical and conservative management.**

    Refer to Clinical recommendations on the use of UAE in the management of fibroids 2013.

20. **(B) 1–2%**

    Refer to Clinical recommendations on the use of UAE in the management of fibroids 2013

    Around 80–90% of patients will be asymptomatic or have significantly improved symptoms at one year with an associated 40–70% reduction in fibroid volume. Hysterectomy may be necessary in up to 2.9% of cases. Early ovarian failure may occur in 1–2%, although this is largely confined to women over 45 or those approaching the menopause. Complications usually occur late (>30 days post-procedure), and may occur >1 year post-procedure.

21. **(E) None**

    Refer to Clinical recommendations on the use of UAE in the management of fibroids 2013.

    The following are absolute contraindications to performing the procedure: Any evidence of current or recent infection in the genital tract Serious doubt as to the diagnosis due to clinical factors or inadequate imaging.

    Asymptomatic fibroids Pregnancy Where a patient would refuse a hysterectomy under any circumstances for social or cultural reasons – even after appropriate counseling that this is necessary after UAE in only a small proportion of cases.

22. **(B) 1–2%**

    Refer to Clinical recommendations on the use of UAE in the management of fibroids 2013.

    A full discussion of complications and their incidence (see Section 10). This should include:
    - Minor complications such as puncture site bruising and self-limiting vaginal discharge (which can occur in 20–30% of patients)
    - Post-embolization syndrome
    - Passage of fibroid material (which may require additional procedures to remove in 6% of patients)

    Permanent amenorrhea (which overall occurs in 1.5–7% of patients Urgent hysterectomy due to infection (in 1% which may occur several months after UAE).

    Patients should be informed that they may require further treatment for recurrent symptoms. The younger they are, the more likely this is. The risk is 25% (by five years) for patients less than 40 years of age and 10% for those between 40 and 50.

23. **(B) 11 per 1,000 pregnancies**

Refer to NICE clinical guidelines 154, December 2012

The rate of ectopic pregnancy is 11 per 1000 pregnancies, with a maternal mortality of 0.2 per 1000 estimated ectopic pregnancies. About two thirds of these deaths are associated with substandard care.

24. **(B) 0.2 per 1,000 pregnancies**

Refer to NICE clinical guidelines 154, December 2012

25. **(D) Recurrent miscarriage**

Refer to NICE clinical guidelines on Ectopic pregnancy and miscarriage September 2014.

26. **(D) Woman with bleeding**

Refer to NICE clinical guidelines on Ectopic pregnancy and miscarriage September 2014

Use expectant management for 7-14 days as the first--line management strategy for women with a confirmed diagnosis of miscarriage. Explore management options other than expectant management if: the woman is at increased risk of hemorrhage (for example, she is in the late first trimester) or she has previous adverse and/or traumatic experience associated with pregnancy (for example, stillbirth, miscarriage or antepartum hemorrhage) or she is at increased risk from the effects of hemorrhage (for example, if she has coagulopathies or is unable to have a blood transfusion) or there is evidence of infection.

27. **(D) Adnexal mass less than 35 mm**

Refer to NICE clinical guidelines on Ectopic pregnancy and miscarriage September 2014

Offer systemic methotrexate as a first-line treatment to women who are able to return for follow-up and who have all of the following: no significant pain an unruptured ectopic pregnancy with an adnexal mass smaller than 35 mm with no visible heartbeat a serum hCG level less than 1500 IU/liter no intrauterine pregnancy (as confirmed on an ultrasound scan).

28. **(D) Haemodynamically stable**

Refer to NICE clinical guidelines on Ectopic pregnancy and miscarriage September 2014

Offer surgery as a first–line treatment to women who are unable to return for follow--up after methotrexate treatment or who have any of the following: an ectopic pregnancy and significant pain an ectopic pregnancy with an adnexal mass of 35 mm or larger an ectopic pregnancy with a fetal heartbeat visible on an ultrasound scan an ectopic pregnancy and a serum hCG level of 5000 IU/liter or more.

29. **(C) 1 in 5**

    Refer to NICE clinical guidelines on Ectopic pregnancy and miscarriage September 2014.

    Inform women having a salpingotomy that up to 1 in 5 women may need further treatment. This treatment may include methotrexate and/or a salpingectomy. Offer a salpingectomy to women undergoing surgery for an ectopic pregnancy unless they have other risk factors for infertility.

30. **(D) Clinical history, USS, laparoscopy and biopsy**

    Refer to ESHRE guidelines on management of Endometriosis 2013.

31. **(B) More than 35 years reduces the change of achieving a pregnancy by 1/10th as compared with paternal age of less than 25 years**

    Refer to TOG 2013

    Assessment of infertile male

    Male age has been shown to have an impact on fertility and offspring health.

    A UK study has shown that paternal age of >35 years halves the chance of achieving a pregnancy compared with a paternal age of <25 years. For this reason, the age of semen donors is limited to 40 or 45 years in some countries.

    Varicoceles, a collection of dilated refluxing veins in the spermatic cord, are found in 11.7% of men with normal semen and 25.4% of men with abnormal semen.

32. **(A) <1%**

    Refer to TOG 2013 Assessment of infertile male

    Hypogonadotrophic hypogonadism is rare and accounts for <1% of male factor fertility problems. It may be congenital or acquired. Causes include craniopharyngiomas, surgery for pituitary tumors, head trauma, hemochromatosis, Kallmann syndrome and other congenital genetic syndromes of reduced gonadotropin releasing hormone (GnRH) secretion (Prader-Willi syndrome, Laurence-Moon-Biedl syndrome).

33. **(C) LH, FSH, Testosterone and prolactin**

    Refer to TOG 2013 Assessment of infertile male

    FSH, LH, testosterone and prolactin should be measured in men with sperm counts of <5 x 106 ml–1. FSH reflects sperm production. Low testosterone levels with high FSH and LH indicate primary testicular failure whereas low testosterone levels in combination with low LH and FSH levels indicate a central defect with secondary hypogonadism.

    A karyotype is indicated in cases of severe oligospermia or azoospermia because these men are at increased risk of structural and sex-- chromosomal anomalies.

34. **(C) 10–15%**

    Refer to TOG 2013 Assessment of infertile male

    As many as 10–15% of men with azoospermia and 5–10% of men with severe oligospermia have underlying micro-deletions in one or more gene regions implicated in spermatogenesis, on the long arm of the Y chromosome (Yq).

35. **(E) All are true**

    Refer to TOG the role of antimullerian hormone as a predictor of ovarian function. 2012

    AMH is a glycoprotein belonging to the transforming growth factor b family. In the male fetus it is expressed in the Sertoli cells of the testes, which leads to mullerian regression. In the female fetus it is expressed by the granulosa cells of the ovary from as early as 36 weeks of gestation and production continues until the menopause. It is expressed mainly by the pre-antral and small antral follicles, declining in dominant follicles and with equivocal expression in atretic follicles, corpus luteum and primordial follicles. AMH is thus a good indicator of the size of the ovarian antral follicle pool. The primary physiological function of AMH in the ovary is inhibition of the recruitment of primordial follicles into the antral follicle pool. AMH also reduces the sensitivity of the growing follicles to FSH.

Practice Question Paper 2

1. **Which statement regarding AMH (Anti-Mullerian hormone) is true?**
   A. High level is suggestive of polycystic ovaries
   B. AMH is a marker of ovarian reserve
   C. It is inferior to FSH and Inhibin B
   D. AMH measurement can help in altering stimulation protocol to prevent/minimize OHSS
   E. All are true

2. **Severe OHSS (ovarian hyper stimulation syndrome) requiring hospitalization is seen in:**
   A. <1%
   B. 1–3%
   C. 5%
   D. 10%
   E. 12–15%

3. **Anti-D prophylaxis for ectopic pregnancy.**
   A. 250 IU of Anti-D is indicated following ectopic pregnancy
   B. 500 IU of Anti-D is indicated
   C. Anti-D is required only for medical management
   D. Anti-D is required only for surgical management
   E. Anti-D not required for ectopic pregnancy

4. **Regarding Anti D which statement is untrue?**
   A. 250 IU of Anti-D prophylaxes is indicated following ectopic pregnancy
   B. 250 IU of Anti-D prophylaxis is indicated between 12 and 20 weeks of gestation following test for feto-maternal hemorrhage (FMH)
   C. Anti-D of 500 IU is indicated within 72 hours of the event after 20 weeks of gestation.
   D. All D negative nonsensitised pregnant women should be offered antenatal prophylaxis with Anti-D at 28 weeks of gestation
   E. All are true

5. **Choose the most appropriate statement. Zidovudine monotherapy can be used in woman planning an elective caesarean section.**
   A. Who has a viral load (VL) of <1000 HIV RNA copies/mL

B. CD4>200 cells/microliter
   C. VL <1000 HIV RNA copies/mL and CD4>200 cells/microlitre
   D. VL <10,000 HIV RNA copies/microliter and CD4>350 cells/microlitre
   E. None

6. **BHIVA guidelines recommendation for ELITE controller:**
   A. Can aim for vaginal delivery
   B. Can aim for breast-feeding
   C. Need not be treated with cART or monotherapy
   D. Should be offered Elective caesarean at 39 weeks of gestation
   E. None are true

7. **Which statement regarding SLE is incorrect?**
   A. More common in men
   B. Usually diagnosed during childbearing years
   C. Antiphospholipid antibody (APA) are present in one-third women with SLE
   D. Women with SLE have two fold increased risk of complications
   E. None

8. **Choose the incorrect statement with regards to SLE.**
   A. SLE flare is more common in second half of pregnancy
   B. Rise in Anti dsDNA titres help to distinguish Pre-eclampsia (PET) from a flare
   C. Definitive investigation to distinguish PET from Lupus nephritis is fall in complement level
   D. Definitive investigation to distinguish PET from Lupus nephritis is renal biopsy
   E. All are correct

9. **Congenital heart block is associated with Anti-Ro/La antibody.**
   A. <1%   B. 2–3%
   C. 5%   D. 15%
   E. 25%

10. **Recurrence of congenital heart block in association with Anti-Ro/La antibody in subsequent pregnancy is:**
    A. 2%   B. 5%
    C. 16%   D. 25%
    E. 50%

11. **Following medication can safely be prescribed in pregnancy in recommended dose and is not associated with congenital anomaly except:**
    A. Corticosteroid   B. Azathioprine
    C. Mycophenolate   D. Ciclosporin
    E. Hydroxychloroquine

12. **Ultrasound feature of ground glass appearance correlates with:**
    A. Hemorrhagic cyst
    B. Hydrosalpinx
    C. Corpus luteal cyst
    D. Endometrioma
    E. Dysgerminoma

13. **Whirl pool sign with reduced vascularity is a ultrasound scan finding specific for:**
    A. Dysgerminoma
    B. Torsion
    C. Corpus luteal cyst
    D. Dermoid
    E. Krukenberg tumor

14. **Most appropriate suture for repair of 3rd degree perineal tear is:**
    A. 2-0 polydioxanone (PDS)
    B. 1-0 Catgut
    C. 2-0 Nylon
    D. 3-0 Monocryl
    E. 3-0 Vicryl

15. **Most common cause of Hirsutism**
    a. Idiopathic
    B. Hyperprolactinemia
    C. Cushing's disease
    D. Polycystic ovary syndrome
    E. Iatrogenic

16. **In _____% of ectopic pregnancy there is normal rise in beta-hCG.**
    A. 1%
    B. 5%
    C. 10%
    D. 15%
    E. 25%

17. **Satellite lesions are seen in:**
    A. *Candida albicans*
    B. Bacterial vaginosis
    C. *Chlamydia trachomatis*
    D. *Trichomonas vaginalis*
    E. Primary syphilis

18. **Choose the correct answer. A term baby dies after a routine forceps delivery.**
    A. Refer to Coroner
    B. Request an inquest
    C. Refer to Coroner: probable postmortem
    D. Refer to GMC
    E. Hospital Postmortem

19. **A woman develops breast cancer and dies at 36 weeks of gestation.**
    A. Direct death
    B. Coincidental death
    C. Indirect death
    D. Nonobstetric death
    E. Pregnancy related death

20. **A woman suffering from postnatal depression kills herself after 40 days of delivery.**
    A. Direct death
    B. Indirect death
    C. Coincidental death
    D. Pregnancy related death
    E. Fortuitous death

21. A previously healthy 22-year-old in her first pregnancy presents at 34 weeks with feeling unwell and shortness of breath (SOB). She develops increasing SOB and died despite intensive resuscitation. Her brother had unexpectedly died at the age of 20 and her chest X ray shows cardiomegaly. Likely cause of death:
    A. Amniotic fluid embolus
    B. Myocardial infarction
    C. Substance Misuse
    D. Pulmonary embolus
    E. Cardiomyopathy

22. A 25-year-old is being induced at 38 weeks of pregnancy for gestational diabetes. She starts contracting within an hour following Prostin, She complains of SOB and collapsed soon and died despite intensive resuscitation. Likely cause of death:
    A. Amniotic fluid embolus
    B. Pulmonary embolus
    C. Myocardial infarction
    D. Cardiovascular Accident (CVA)
    E. Cardiomyopathy

23. *Listeria* in pregnancy is associated with all except:
    A. Miscarriage and preterm delivery
    B. Meconium stained liquor
    C. Multiple abscess and granuloma in lung, liver and brain
    D. Associated with intake of soft cheese
    E. Associated with obstetric cholestasis

24. Features of a baby born with HIV are all except:
    A. Strawberry head
    B. Square box like forehead
    C. Patulous wide set eyes
    D. All are true
    E. None

25. Celery stalk femur is associated with:
    A. HIV
    B. Toxoplasmosis
    C. Rubella
    D. Syphilis
    E. Echovirus

26. A woman presents at 28 weeks of gestation with sudden onset of severe headache, describing as worst headache ever. Her BP is 124/78 mm Hg and urine dip –NAD. Likely diagnosis is:
    A. Tension headache
    B. Sub-arachnoid
    C. Migraine
    D. Meningitis
    E. Cluster headache

27. A woman presents with headache along with pain poking in the eye along with lacrimation and running nose.
    A. Tension headache
    B. Sub-arachnoid
    C. Migraine
    D. Meningitis
    E. Cluster headache

28. Breastfeeding is contraindicated in following except:
    A. Active untreated tuberculosis
    B. Galactosemia
    C. Maternal intake of Lithium
    D. All
    E. None

29. **Feature of Prune belly syndrome is:**
    A. Congenital disorder of urinary system
    B. Congenital absence of abdominal muscles
    C. Commonly seen in males
    D. Ultrasound scan shows large abdominal cavity and distended bladder
    E. All

30. **Which condition is incorrectly paired?**
    A. Potter syndrome—Kidney
    B. Anencephaly—Forebrain
    C. Prune belly syndrome—Urinary tract
    D. Arnold Chiari malformation—Kidney
    E. Turner syndrome—Ovary

31. **Choose the USS feature that is incorrectly paired:**
    A. Lemon sign—Cerebellum
    B. Echogenic bowel—Cystic fibrosis
    C. Double bubble sign—Duodenal atresia
    D. Lambda sign—Monochorionic twins
    E. All are correct

32. **Nerves affected in Erb's palsy.**
    A. C5
    B. C6
    C. C8
    D. C8–T1
    E. C5–C6

33. **Risk of perforation during Evacuation in second trimester is around:**
    A. 0.1%
    B. 1%
    C. 5%
    D. 10%
    E. 25%

34. **Reduced liquor seen in following except:**
    A. Potter syndrome
    B. Prune belly syndrome
    C. Rubella
    D. All
    E. None

35. **Polymorphic eruptions of pregnancy:**
    A. More common in third trimester and immediate postpartum.
    B. Risk factors include nulliparity, multiple pregnancy and overdistension
    C. Erythematous papules are located within the abdominal striae
    D. There is periumbilical sparing
    E. There is high recurrence in subsequent pregnancy

36. **Chronic nerve related pain following Pfannenstiel incision is usually due to involvement of:**
    A. Ilioinguinal nerve
    B. Iliohypogastric nerve
    C. Genitofemoral nerve
    D. Lateral cutaneous nerve
    E. Ilioinguinal and Iliohypogastric nerve

ANSWERS

1. **(C) It is inferior to FSH and Inhibin B**

   Refer to TOG 2012 "The role of anti – mullerian hormone as a predictor of ovarian function".

   Ovarian reserve may not always match chronological age, leading to deviations from the normogram. These variations may be due to genetic, autoimmune or environmental factors and may or may not be reversible. Decreased AMH levels are indicative of a reduced antral follicle pool and hence reduced ovarian reserve, independent of age. High levels of AMH are suggestive of polycystic ovaries. AMH is shown to be comparable to antral follicle count as a marker of ovarian reserve, but is superior to FSH and inhibin B.

2. **(B) 1–3%**

   Refer to TOG 2012 the role of anti – mullerian hormone as a predictor of ovarian function.

   Between 15–20% of women undergoing controlled ovarian hyper-stimulation for IVF have mild to moderate ovarian hyperstimulation syndrome (OHSS) and 1–3% have severe OHSS requiring hospitalisation

3. **(A) 250 IU of anti-D is indicated following ectopic pregnancy**

   British Committee for standards in Hematology (BCSH) guidelines for the use of Anti-D immunoglobulin for the prevention of the hemolytic disease of the fetus and the newborn. 2014

   In pregnancies less than 12 weeks gestation, Anti-D Ig G prophylaxis is only indicated following ectopic pregnancy, molar pregnancy, therapeutic termination of pregnancy, and in cases of uterine bleeding where this is repeated, heavy or associated with abdominal pain. The minimum dose should be 250 IU. A test for FMH is not required.

4. **(B) 250 IU of Anti-D is indicated between 12 and 20 weeks of gestation following FMH**

   Refer to (BCSH) guidelines for the use of Anti-D immunoglobulin for the prevention of the hemolytic disease of the fetus and the newborn. 2014.

5. **(D) VL<10,000 HIV RNA copies/microlitre and CD 4>350 cells/microlitre**

   Refer to BHIVA-pregnancy guidelines 2014.

   Untreated women with a CD4 cell count ≥350 cells/μL and a viral load of <50 HIV RNA copies/mL (confirmed on a separate assay): can be treated with zidovudine monotherapy or with cART (including abacavir/lamivudine/zidovudine).

Zidovudine monotherapy can be used in women planning a caesarean section who have a baseline VL of < 10 000 HIV RNA copies/mL and a CD4 of > 350 cells/μ L.

6. **(A) Can aim for vaginal delivery**

   Refer to BHIVA-pregnancy guidelines 2014.

   Untreated women with a CD4 cell count ≥ 350 cells/μL and a viral load of < 50 HIV RNA copies/mL (confirmed on a separate assay): can be treated with zidovudine monotherapy or with cART (including abacavir/lamivudine/zidovudine). Can aim for a vaginal delivery. Should exclusively formula feed their infant.

7. **(A) More common in men**

   Reference: TOG 2012 SLE volume 14 Maternal and Fetal complications of SLE. Systemic lupus erythematosus (SLE) is an idiopathic autoimmune condition, which has multi-organ involvement. The disease affects women and men in a ratio of 10:1.

   More commonly affects Afro-Caribbean than Asian population. Most women seem to be diagnosed during the childbearing years. The prevalence of SLE in women of childbearing years is around 1 in 500.

8. **(C) Definitive investigation to distinguish PET from Lupus nephritis is fall in Complement level**

   Refer to TOG 2012 volume 14 "Maternal and Fetal complications of SLE"

   The risk of an SLE flare in pregnancy is increased with active disease in the 3–6 months prior to conception, with the majority of flares occurring in the second half of pregnancy.

   Distinguishing Pre-eclampsia from Lupus nephritis is perhaps, the most challenging aspect of obstetric management. The features of lupus nephritis include hypertension and proteinuria with or without hematuria and renal impairment.

   The presence of hematuria or red cell casts as well as a rise in anti-dsDNA titres or a fall in complement levels help to distinguish this from pre-eclampsia; in addition, lupus disease activity in non-renal organ systems suggests that a lupus nephritis flare is more likely.

9. **(B) 2–3%**

   Refer to TOG 2012 volume 14 "Maternal and Fetal complications of SLE"

   Congenital heart block is associated with maternal anti-Ro/La autoantibodies. Antibodies cross the placenta and destroy the Purkinje system. The usual presentation is a fixed fetal bradycardia of 60–80 beats per minute on ultrasound scan. It occurs in 2–3% of fetuses of women with the anti-Ro/La antibody and there is a recurrence rate of 16% in subsequent pregnancies. It is associated with significant perinatal morbidity and mortality, with about half of infants requiring pacing by the first year of life. Congenital heart block develops between 18–28 weeks of gestation and fetal echocardiography should be performed around this period to detect it.

10. **(C) 16%**

    Refer to TOG 2012 volume 14 "Maternal and Fetal complications of SLE". Same as above.

11. **(C) Mycophenolate**

    Refer to TOG 2012 volume 14 "Maternal and Fetal complications of SLE"

    Glucocorticoids, mainly in the form of prednisolone, are frequently but not exclusively used as one of the first-line treatments in pregnancy. The dosage used does not vary greatly between pregnant and non-pregnant patients. The risk of adverse effects of steroids on the fetus is thought to be low, with little evidence for congenital malformations or neonatal adrenal suppression. Other immunosuppressant agents that are frequently used and are generally considered safe during pregnancy include azathioprine and hydroxychloroquine. There is no indication to discontinue them during pregnancy. It is also worth noting that several drugs can cause a lupus-like syndrome. The most common of these are: Hydralazine, procainamide, quinidine, isoniazid, diltiazem and minocycline.

12. **(D) Endometrioma**

    Ultrasound in Obstetrics and gynecology: A practical approach.

13. **(B) Torsion**

    Ultrasound in Obstetrics and gynecology: A practical approach.

14. **(A) 2-0 PDS**

    Refer to RCOG GTG No. 29 June 2015.

    3-0 polyglactin should be used to repair the anorectal mucosa as it may cause less irritation and discomfort than polydioxanone (PDS) sutures. When repair of the EAS and/or IAS muscle is being performed, either monofilament sutures such as 3-0 PDS or modern braided sutures such as 2-0 polyglactin can be used with equivalent outcomes.

    When obstetric anal sphincter repairs are being performed, the burying of surgical knots beneath the superficial perineal muscles is recommended to minimise the risk of knot and suture migration to the skin.

15. **(A) Idiopathic**

    Refer to TOG 2009

    Hirsutism in young women. Hirsutism is the presence of terminal (course) hairs in females in a male like pattern. Affects 5-15% of the women. The causes can be broadly divided into Androgen excess, Non-androgen factors and Idiopathic.

    Androgen causes-PCOS, Androgen secreting tumors. Non classic CAH.

Non Androgen causes–Factors with unknown mechanism of action on hair follicles like drugs (Phenytoin. Minoxidil, Diazoxide, Streptomycin, high dose corticosteroid) Idiopathic-6–7%.

16. **(D) 15%**

    Refer to TOG July 2014.

17. **(A)** *Candida Albicans*

    Refer to TOG October 2001 "Management of recurrent vulvovaginal candidiasis" There is also erythema, fissures along with satellite lesions. The vaginal pH is <4.5. The bacterial vaginosis there is vaginal redness, blood stained discharge and Clue cells. Often they are cyclical and get worse during menses and vaginal pH >4.5.

18. **(C) Refer to Coroner: Probable postmortem**

19. **(B) Coincidental Death**

    Refer to MBRRACE

20. **(B) Indirect death**

    Refer to MBRRACE

21. **(E) Cardiomyopathy**

    Refer to MBRRACE and (ESC) Guidelines on the management of cardiovascular diseases during pregnancy 2011.

22. **(A) Amniotic fluid embolus**

    Refer to MBRRACE and European society of cardiologists (ESC) Guidelines on the management of cardiovascular diseases during pregnancy. 2011.

23. **(E) Associated with obstetric cholestasis**

    Refer to Listeriosis in pregnancy (NHS choices/BabyCenter)

    Listeriosis is an illness caused by a bacteria found in certain foods, in soil or in animal poo. The scientific name for the bacteria is listeria monocytogenes, or listeria for short.

    But it's worth remembering that listeriosis is rare, even in pregnant women. There are fewer than 200 cases in the UK each year, and fewer than 30 of these cases are pregnant women.

    When a pregnant woman has listeriosis, the infection may be passed on to her baby in the womb or during birth. However, without treatment, listeriosis can sometimes have serious consequences. Sadly, untreated listeriosis can lead to: Miscarriage, premature birth and stillbirth.

24. **(A) Strawberry head**

    Refer to HIV in children and Infants.

    HIV infection is often difficult to diagnose in very young children. Infected babies, especially in the first few months of life, often appear normal and may exhibit no telltale signs that would allow a definitive diagnosis of HIV infection. Moreover, all children born to infected mothers have antibodies to HIV, made by the mother's immune system, that cross the placenta to the baby's bloodstream before birth and persist for up to 18 months. Because these maternal antibodies reflect the mother's but not the infant's infection status, the test is not useful in newborns or young infants.

About 20 percent of children develop serious disease in the first year of life; most of these children die by age 4 years. The remaining 80 percent of infected children have a slower rate of disease progression, many not developing the most serious symptoms of AIDS until school entry or even adolescence.

25. **(D) Syphilis**

    Other features associated with Rubella are Cataract, Deafness, Heart abnormalities (Patent ductus arteriosus) and brain damage.

26. **(B) Sub-arachnoid**

    Refer to TOG 2014 volume 16.

    Headaches are common in pregnancy, most are benign like migraine and tension-type headache but pregnant women are at risk of life threatening secondary headaches like impending eclampsia and cerebral venous thrombosis. Failure to recognise potentially devastating conditions can lead to increased maternal morbidity and mortality.

27. **(E) Cluster headache**

    Refer to TOG 2014

    Migraine gets worse with activity, usually unilateral and gradually increasing in intensity.

    Tension headache is temporal in site. Meningitis has neck stiffness. Cluster headache is a rare type of headache that affects about 1 to 2 people in every 1,000. It is one of the most painful conditions an individual can experience, described as excruciating and even more debilitating than migraine.

    The symptoms of cluster headache are very typical. The pain in the head is always unilateral (one sided), although for some people the side can vary from time to time. The pain is usually centered over one eye, one temple or the forehead.

    During a bout of cluster headache the pain is often experienced at a similar time each day. The headache often starts at night waking people one to two hours after they have gone to sleep. The pain usually reaches its full intensity within 5 to 10 minutes and lasts at this agonizing level for between 30 and 60 minutes. For some people the pain can last for 15 minutes, for others 3 hours has been known. It then stops, usually fairly abruptly. In about 80% of people with cluster headache the bouts (or "clusters") of head pain last for 4 to 12 weeks once a year often at the same time and often in the spring or autumn.

28. **(D) All**

Breastfeeding may not be in best interest of the baby in the following conditions:
- The baby has Galactosaemia
- Mother has active untreated tuberculosis, T-cell lymphotrophic virus type 1 or 2.
- Mother is receiving diagnostic or therapeutic radio-active isotopes or has had exposure to radioactive materials
- Mother is receiving antimetabolites or other chemotherapeutic agents
- Mother is abusing drugs
- Mother has herpes simplex lesions on a breast (the baby may feed from the other breast if free from lesions)
- Mother is HIV positive.

29. **(E) All**

Prune belly syndrome is a group of birth defects that involve three main problems:
- Poor development of the abdominal muscles, causing the skin of the belly area to wrinkle like a prune.
- Undescended testicles (cryptorchidism).
- Urinary tract problems

The causes of prune belly syndrome are unknown. The condition affects mostly boys.
- Weak abdominal muscles can cause:
- "Little Buddha" appearance
- Constipation
- Delay in sitting and walking
- Difficulties coughing

Urinary tract problems can cause difficulty urinating.

30. **(D) Arnold Chiari Malformation—Kidney**

In Arnold Chiari malformation the brain is affected

31. **(D) Lamda sign—Monochorionic Twins**

The scan feature for Monochorionic twins is T-sign whereas Dichorionic twins show Twin Peak sign or Lambda sign.

32. **(E) C5–C6**

Refer to TOG 2014 Number 1

The upper brachial plexus is affected in Erb's palsy and involves C5 and C6.

Erb's palsy causes inability to abduct the shoulder, externally rotate the arm and supinate the forearm. This deformity is also called "Porter's tip hand Klumpke's palsy affects C8–T1 (Lower Brachial plexus) and is much less common than Erb's palsy and has poor prognosis.

33. **(C) 5%**

    TOG 2013 Number 4.

    Factors that increase the risk of uterine perforation include uterine anomalies, infection, recent pregnancy and postmenopause. TOP is the most common procedure associated with uterine perforation. Gynecologists (RCOG) on best practice in outpatient hysteroscopy suggest an average incidence of perforation of 0.002–1.7%. Most perforations are in the body of the uterus and are often small tending to cause relatively little hemorrhage. The site of perforation that is most common is the anterior wall of the uterus.

34. **(D) All**

35. **(E) There is high recurrence in subsequent pregnancy.**

    Refer to TOG 2013 Number 4.

36. **(E) Ilioinguinal and Iliohypogastric nerve**

    Refer to TOG 2014 Number 1.